KDP amazon

Middle third fracture

[Document subtitle]

Dr, Adil Sulieman
8-4-2023

The middle third facial bones fracture

Dr ADIL SULEMAN MOHAMMED

Copy right ISBN.

9798388276315

Panda face and raccoon eye appears in Lefort 2 and 3 but

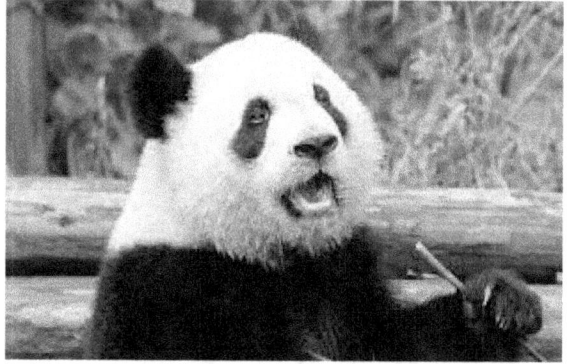

Panda face in Lefort 3 commonly

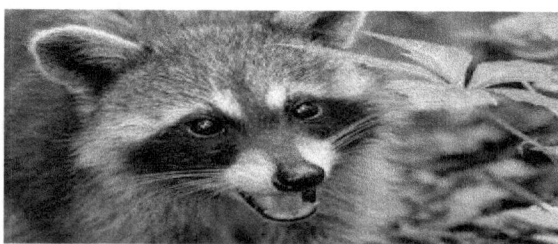

Raccoon eyes in Lefort 2

ACKNOWDEGEMENT

To my great family

To my darling wife Dr Shiraz, the great beloved dentist who tolerate me.

To my great brother Dr Mamoun, the great and brilliant dentist who gave his advice.

To my nice and beautiful girls

Ghina, Muna, Hoor and the little one Ragad

Godless them.

To my great professors and teachers and my friends

To my daughter the brilliant drawer Muna, she helps me.

In making drawing in this book.

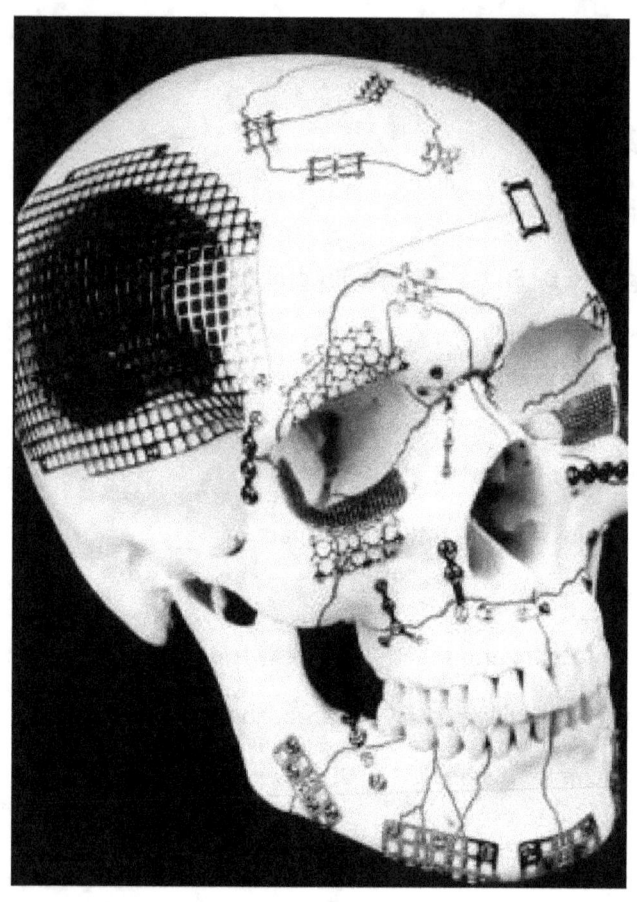

Figure 1 Different methods of Facial bone fracture fixation

Table of Contents

The middle third fracture

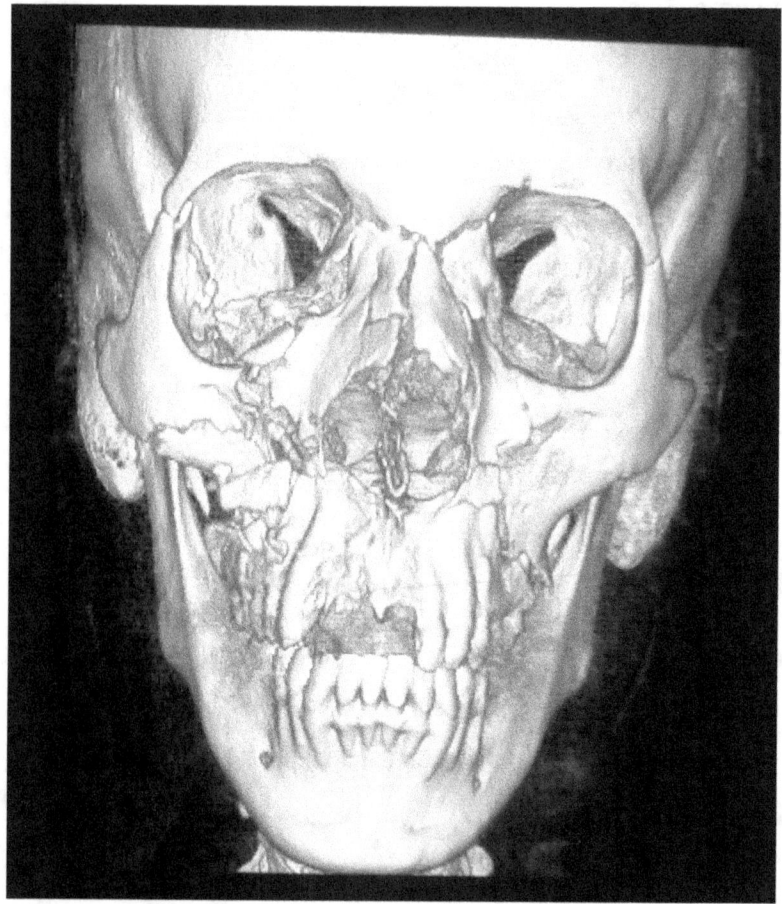

Figure 3DCT Facial bone showing middle third facial bone fractures.

Preface

This topic is small gift which had been written with golden words to any student and dentist who respect the science and respect their teachers .my grate thankfulness and respect extended to my teaches in oral and maxillofacial surgery department in Khartoum (Sudan) dental teaching hospital without them, I did not know this information.

This is clinical notes about the middle third facial bone fracture., clinical features and radiology and treatment also helpful questions and answer, this book can be using as small reference for dental students and maxillofacial surgeon.

This book is small drop in the ocean of maxillofacial surgeon.

Chapter one
Illustrate Mqs

1. During you do GCS assessment if the pt get his hand flex to his body figure 1
   This position is: _

A. Prone position

B. Decorticate position.

C. Decerebrate position

D. all the above

The correct answer is B.

Manifestations of Brain Injury

Decorticate posturing

Decerebrate posturing

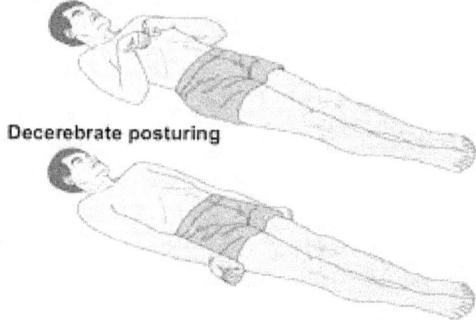

Figure 1

2.In GCS the abnormal extension decerebrate position

   A. Is score 3 in M motor.
   B. Is score 2 in M motor.

C. Is score 5 in M motor.

D. None of 1 in M motor.

The correct answer is B.

3. If the GCS the 15 scores are

A.E4, V5, M6.

B. E4, V6, M5.

C.M4, E5, V6.

D. E3, V6, M5.

The correct answer is A

4.If the GCS is 4 the condition of the patient

A. Mild

B. Moderate.

C. Sever.

D. it is OK.

The correct answer is C.

Behaviour	Response
Eye Opening Response	4. Spontaneously 3. To speech 2. To pain 1. No response
Verbal Response	5. Oriented to time, person and place 4. Confused 3. Inappropriate words 2. Incomprehensible sounds 1. No response
Motor Response	6. Obeys command 5. Moves to localised pain 4. Flex to withdraw from pain 3. Abnormal flexion 2. Abnormal extension 1. No response

Table 1 Glasco coma scale (GCS)

5.In case of PA Skull view one answer is correct

    A. The x-ray beam come the behind the patient.
    B. The x-ray beam come the front of the patient.
    C. It is Towne view.
    D. It is Submentovertex view.

The correct answer is A

The x-ray beam it is straight from behind.

The skull posteroanterior (PA) view is a non-angled radiograph of the skull.

X-ray detector

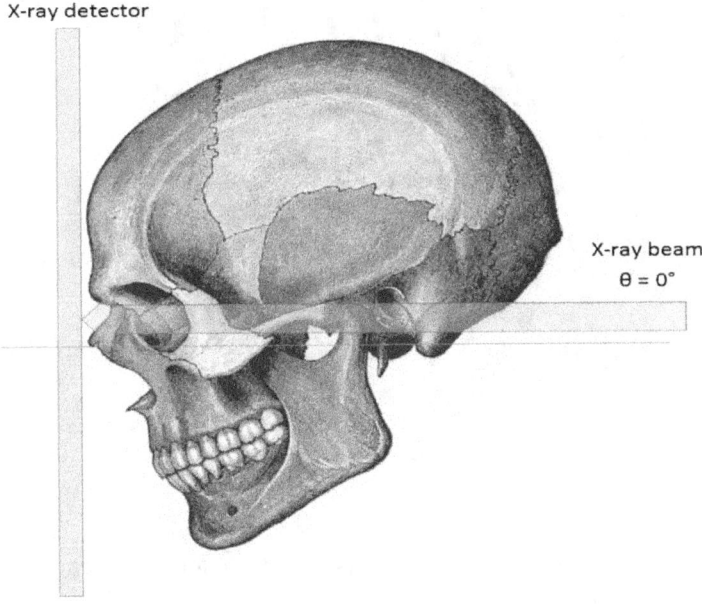

X-ray beam
θ = 0°

Figure 2 showing PA skull view.

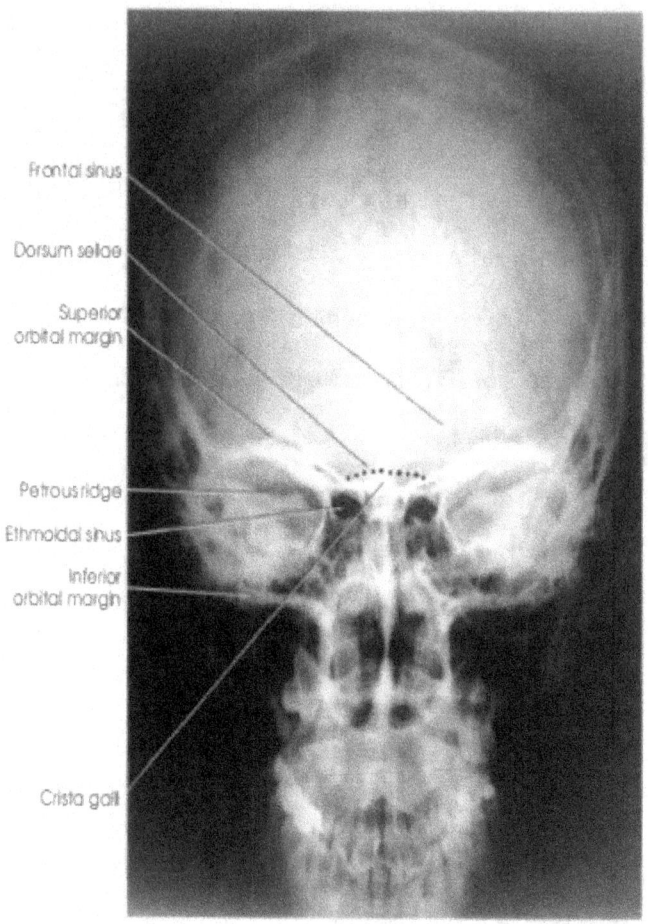

Figure 3 PA skull view

The skull anteroposterior (AP) view is a non-angled radiograph of the skull. This view provides an overview of the entire skull rather than attempting to highlight any one region.

The x-ray beam it is straight from front.

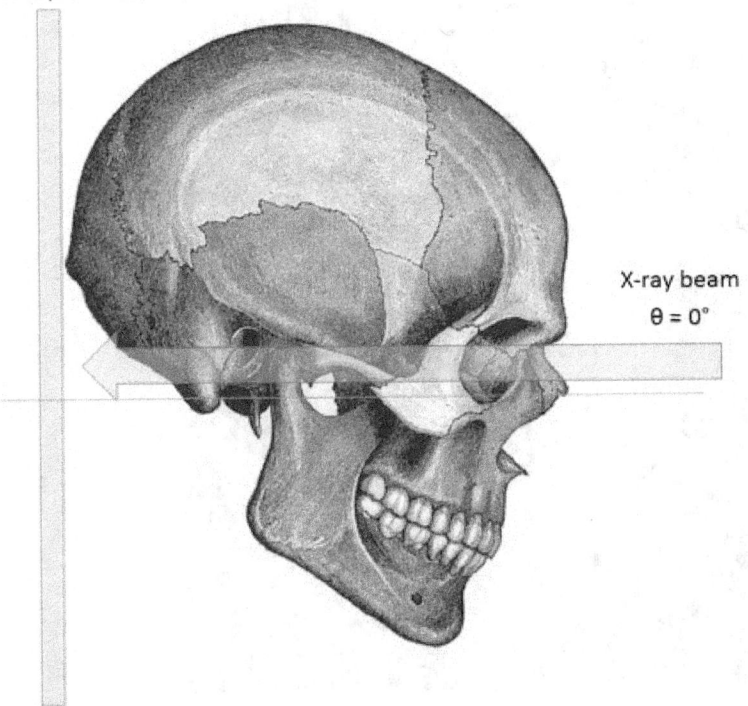

X-ray detector

X-ray beam
θ = 0°

Figure 4 showing the beam of AP skull view.

6.The Towne view is.

A.30degree lateral skull view

B. 30-degree AP view

C. 30-degree PA view

D. None of the above

The correct answer is C.

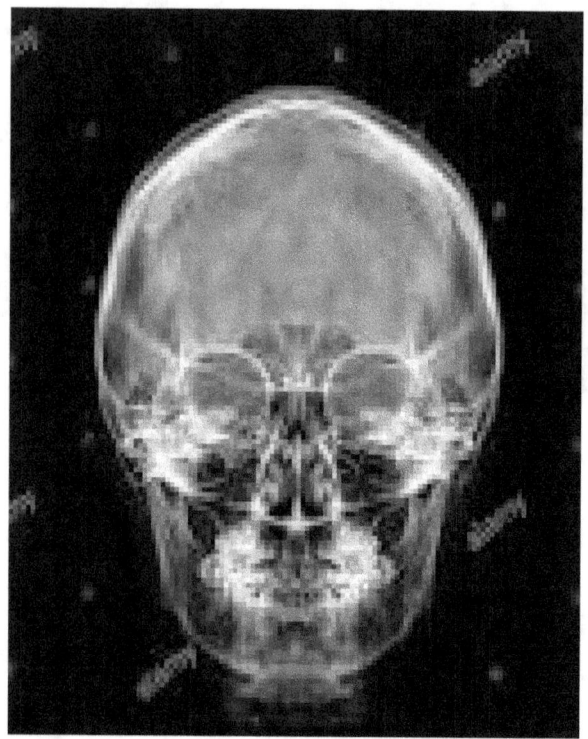

Figure 5 the Towne view

The Towne view is an angled anteroposterior radiograph of the skull and visualizes the petrous part of the pyramids, the dorsum sellae and the posterior clinoid processes. which are visible in the shadow of the foramen magnum.

It 30-degree PA view

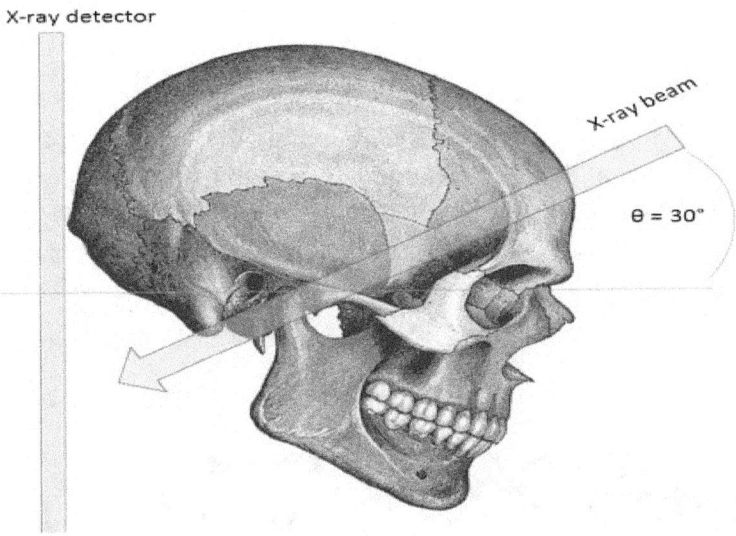

X-ray detector

X-ray beam

θ = 30°

Figure 6 the water view beam 30 degree

7.Another name for water view is: -

A. Occipitomental view

B. Submentovertex view

C. lateral skull view

D.PA Skull view

8.The water view (occipitomental view) best view is showing.

A The maxillary sinus

B. The fracture condyle

C. the symphysis fracture

D. None of the above

Waters' view (also known as the occipitomental view) is a radiographic view of the skull. It is commonly used to get a better view of the maxillary sinuses. An x-ray beam is angled at 45° to the orbitomeatal line. The rays pass from behind the head and are perpendicular to the radiographic plate.

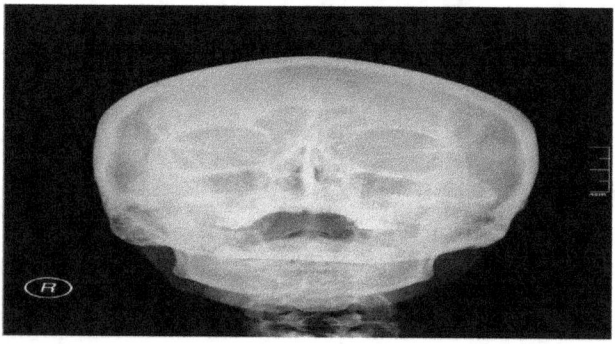

The figure7 shows the water view or occipitomental view.

9.The Submentovertex view is best view for

    A.   Fracture condyle of the mandible
    B.   Frontal bone fracture
    C.   The zygomatic arch fractures.
    D.   None of the above

the correct answer is C.

The skull Submentovertex view is an angled anterosuperior radiograph of the base of skull. As this view involves radiographic positioning that is uncomfortable for the patient and with CT being more sensitive to bony detail, this view is rapidly becoming obsolete.

10.In the Submentovertex view

A. The x-ray beam come from the vertex of the skull.

B. The x-ray beam come lower border of the mandible.

C, it is Towne view.

D. None of the above.

The correct answer is B.

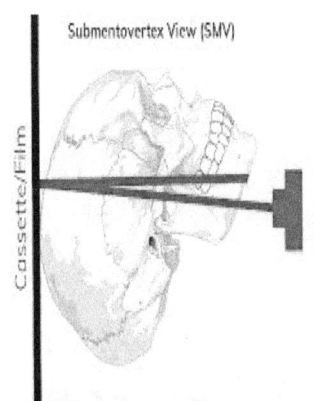

The figure 8 showing beam of Submentovertex.

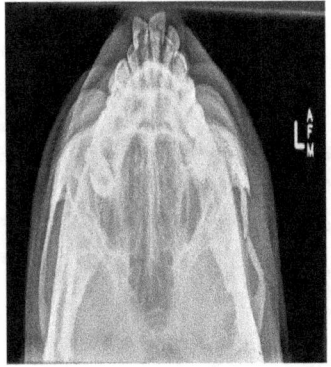

The figure 9 showing Submentovertex view.

11.If the patient did MRI view for the brain

Showing this view, the CSF is white. In figure 10

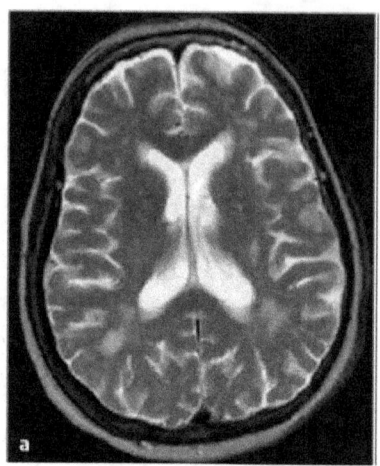

Figure 10

    A. Is Flair view of MRI brain.
    B. It is T1 phase of MRI Brain.
    C. It is T2 phase OF MRI brain.
    D. None of the above

The correct answer is C.

there are different contrast images in magnetic resonance MRI types. T1-weighted MRI enhances the signal of the fatty tissue and suppresses the signal of the water. T2-weighted MRI enhances the signal of the water.

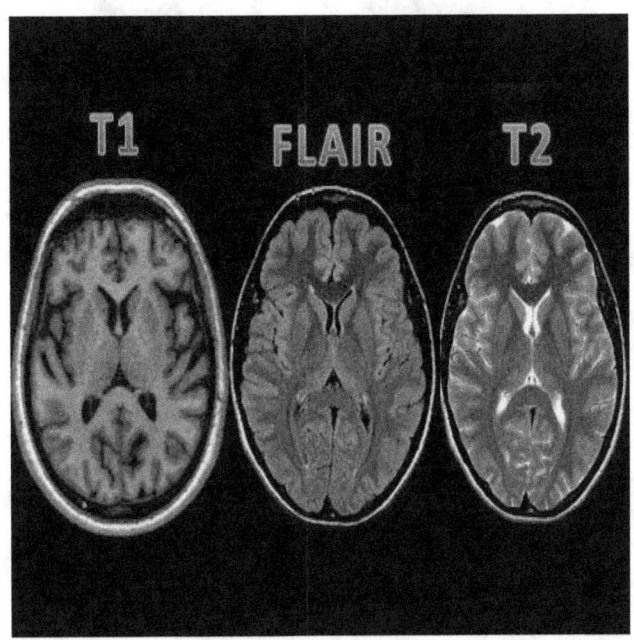

Figure 11 Magnetic resonance image différent phases

T1		T2
Darker	Gray matter	Lighter
Lighter	White matter	Darker
Dark	CSF	White
White	Fat	Less white

Table 2 showing the different between MRI t1.T2 phases

12.IF CT brain done for patient has craniofacial injury it is showing

This view in this CT brain figure 12 showing.

A. It is epidural hemorrhage.

B. It is subdural hemorrhage.

C. Its subarachnoid hemorrhage.

Figure 12

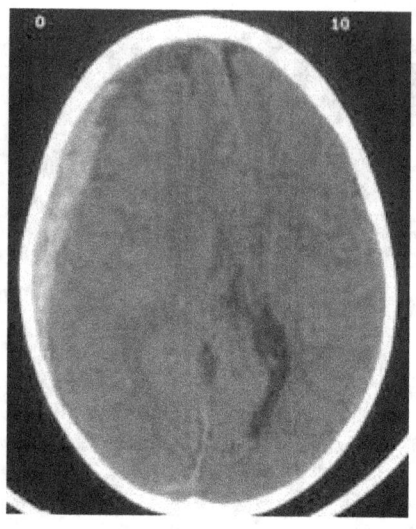

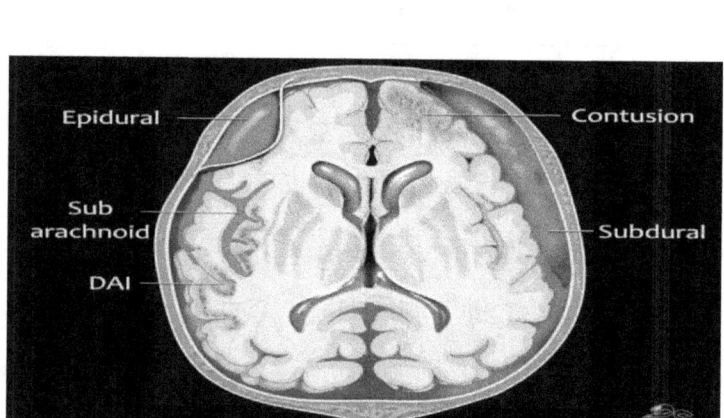

Figure 13 showing different types of brain hemorrhage.

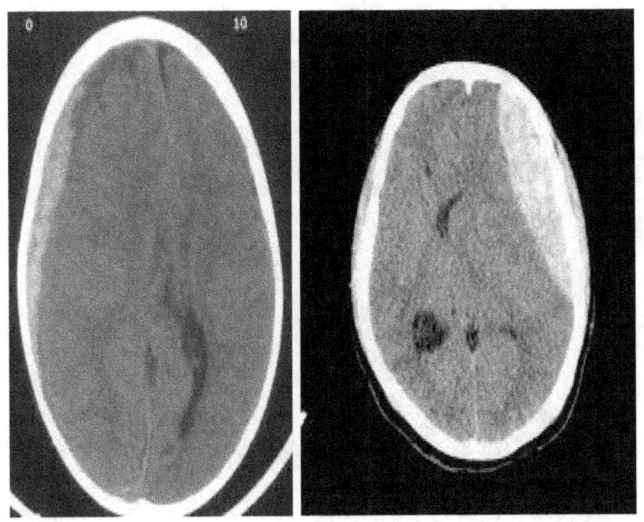

Figure 14,15

fSubdural hamorrhage   epidural hamorrhage

Subdural hamorrhage	epidural hamorrhage
Concave -cresent shape	Convex – lens shape
Bridge vein	Middle meningeal artery
Eldery -alcoholic	Lucid interval

Table 3 The different between subdural and epidural hemorrhage

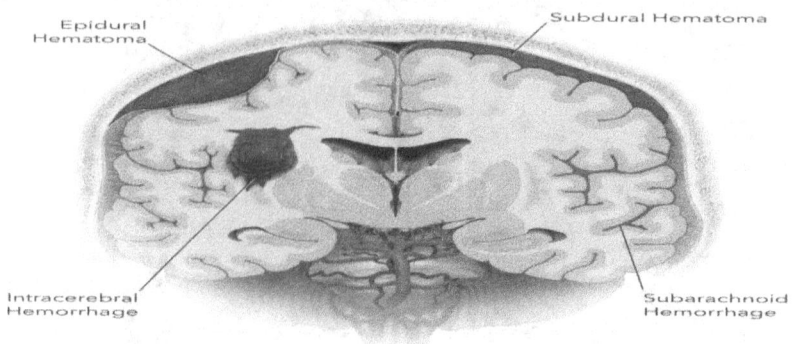

Figure 16 showing intracerbral and subarachnoid hemorrhage

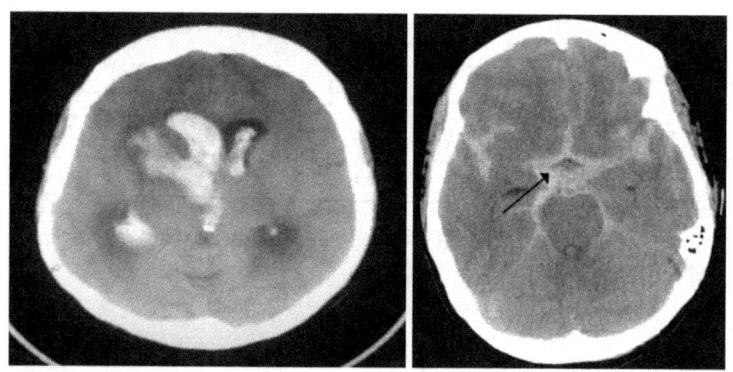

Figure 17,18

Intracerbral haemmorhge   subarahnoid haemmorhge

13.Dish face deformity

   A. It occurs in lefort 3 fracture
   B. The face is concave in shape
   C. It is occur in craniofacial disjuction

21

D.   All of the above

The correct answer is D

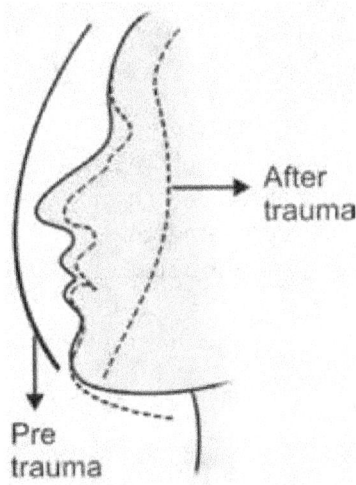

After
trauma

Pre
trauma

Figure 19 showing dish face after trauma

14.In case of facial truma you doublt about CSF leakage

In handkershief the patient show this sign which indicated CSF leakkage

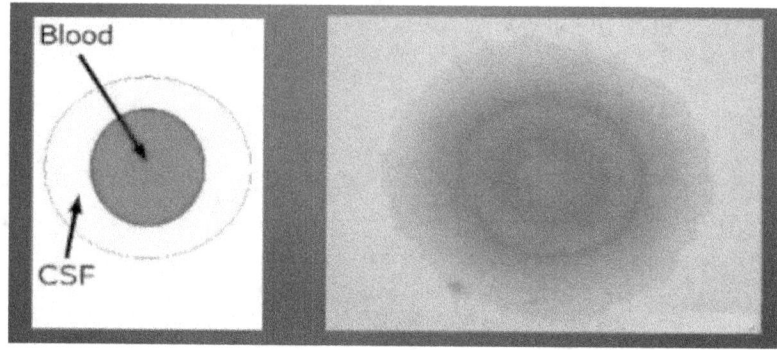

A. figure 20
B. It is double hallow sign.
C. It is battle sign.
D. It is guern sign.
E. Tear drop sign.

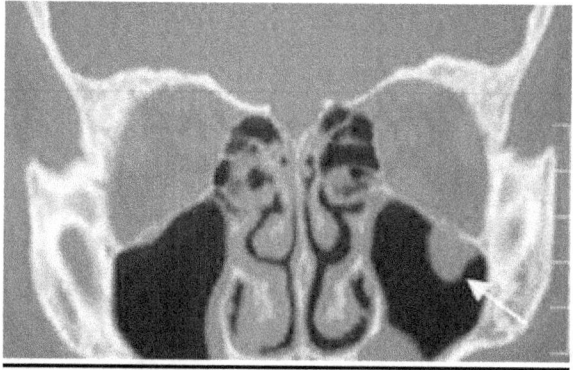

F. Figure 21
Tear drop sign for blow out fracture.

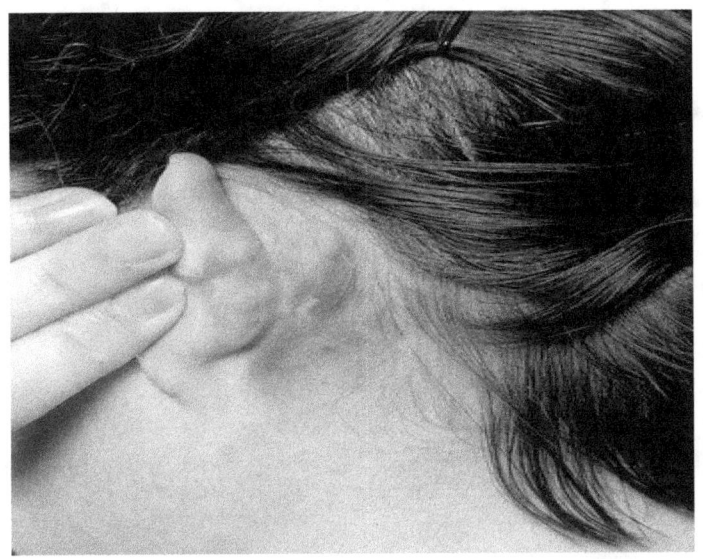

Figure 22 Battle sign base of skull fracture

15.Circumorbital ecchymosis is found all except
A. Lefort 1
B. Lefort 3
c. Zygomatic bone fracture
D. Blow out fracture.

The correct answer is A
Because in Lefort 1 fracture the orbit not involved.

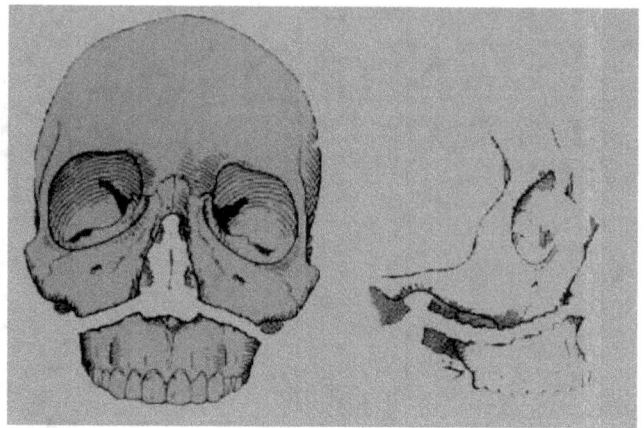

Figure 31
Lefort 1 fracture the orbit not involved.

16. During eye examination one eye is smaller than other
This condition is called.
- A. Strabismus
- B. Dipoplia
- C. Squint
- D. Anisocoria

The correct answer is D.
Strabismus is squint that occur by abducent nerve, the six cranial nerve involvement the eye cannot look laterally, it is isotropia.
The affected eye looks medially.

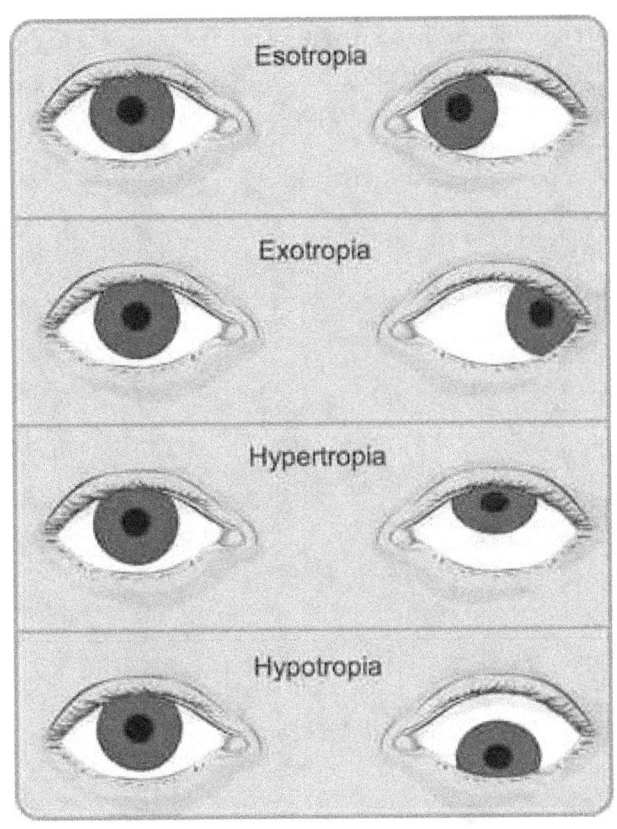

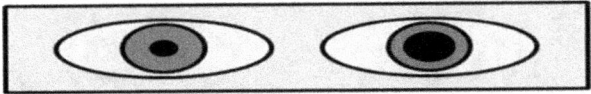

Anisocoria
Right pupil does not have the same size as left pupil

Figure 23,24

17.If both eye dilated fixed it sign of
   A.   Loss of conscious or
   GCS is 3
   B. both eye mydriasis
   C. May be sign of brain death.
   D.   All of the above

the correct answer is D

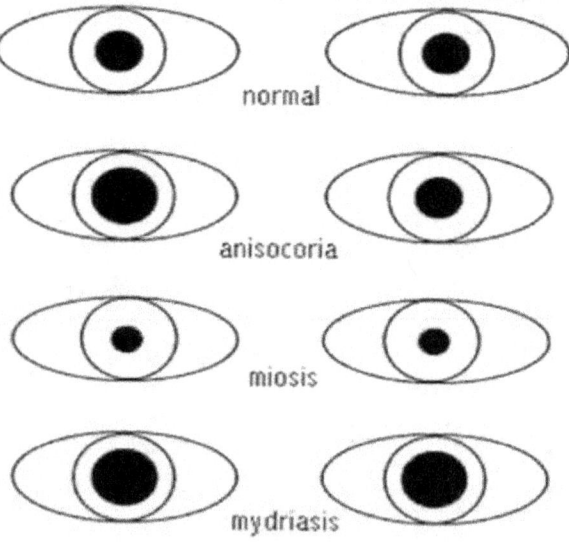

normal

anisocoria

miosis

mydriasis

Figure 25 showing different eye sizes

Chapter Two
Introduction

Traumatology

In head and neck trauma

The neck can divide in different zones.

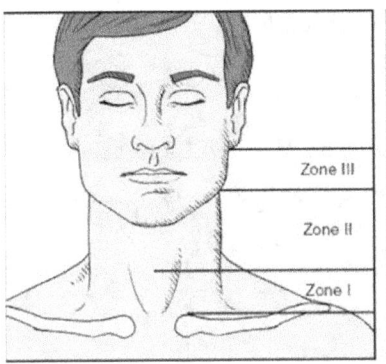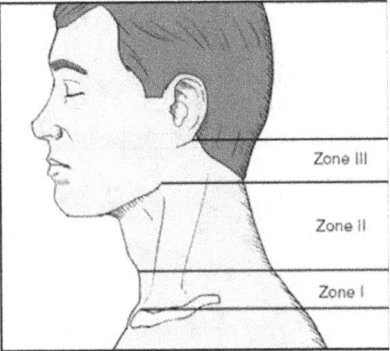

Figure 26 showing **different neck zones.**

Zone1 It is located between the clavicle and hyoid bone.

Zone 2 it is located between the hyoid bone and angle of the mandible.

Zone 3 between the angle of the mandible to the Mastoid bone (base of skull)

The traumatology

Defined as the science which concern particularly with study of trauma, fracture, and injury.

The word fracture means breakage and discontinuity of bone fragments.

The facial skeleton

The facial skeleton is divided into.

1.The upper third which extend form the cranium to the level from bilateral frontozygomatic suture and extended to frontonasal suture.

2. The middle third fracture from the bilateral frontozygomatic suture to the level of maxilla

3. The lower third which form the mandible

The surgical anatomy

The bones constituting the middle third facial bone fracture.

The bones of the skull and face collectively makeup the most complex area of the facial skeletons is (Figure27)

1. The maxillae.
2. The palatine bones.
3. The zygomatic bones
4. Temporal process of zygomatic bone.
5. The nasal bone.
6. The lacrimal bone.
7. The ethmoid one and attached conchae.
8. The inferior conchae.
9. The pterygoid plate of sphenoid bone.
10. The vomer.

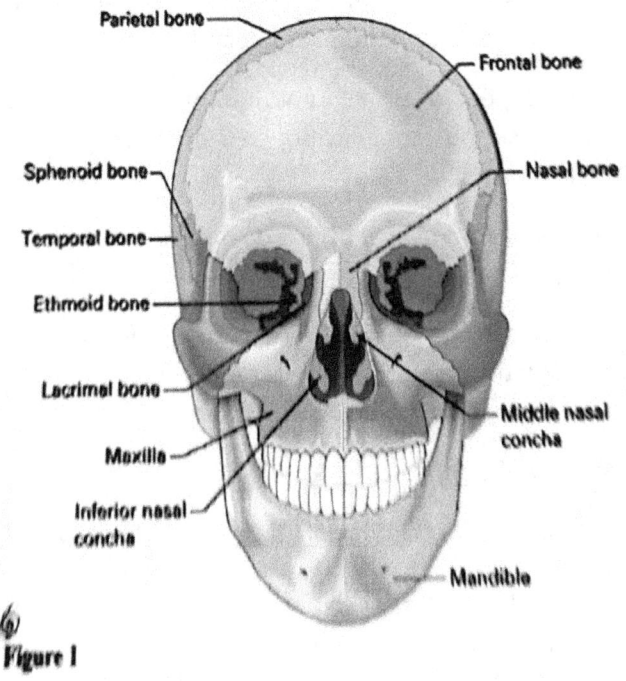

Parietal bone

Frontal bone

Sphenoid bone

Nasal bone

Temporal bone

Ethmoid bone

Lacrimal bone

Middle nasal concha

Maxilla

Inferior nasal concha

Mandible

Figure 1

Figure 27 middle third facial bones

Why we study the middle third facial bone fracture.

The middle third of the facial skeleton

1. Provide protection of the brain and cranial nerves
2. Prevent respiratory obstruction.

30

3. Prevent bleeding by saving the blood vessels.
4. Preservation of life
5. Maintenance of function
6. Restoration of the appearance (aesthetics)

the mortality rates have three peaks: -

1.The first peak mortality within seconds or minutes due to vital structure injury (the brain and heart).

2. The second peak occur in some minutes to hours due to unrecognized serious complications such as ventilatory and haemorrhage.

3.The third peak is mortality occurs days to several weeks due to multiorgan failure.

The first peak is not amenable to secondary preventive measurement by active professional intervention like the second peak is prevented by patient resuscitation.

The aetiology of trauma

The causes of middle third facial injury it could be divided to

 a) Direct injury.

b) Indirect injury (coup injury) (Figure28)

1. Direct injury or violence (assault) it is threat or interpersonal altercation or fight e.g., Fist fighting or boxing.
2. Road traffic accident (RTA) nowadays is the commonest cause of trauma due to civilization and alcohol drinking in many countries it could be prevented by wearing safety seat belt, increase policing, increase traffic light, crumpling zone, collapsing steering wheels, antilock braking system, laminated wind screen and airbag, wearing of helmets crash in motorcycle.

3. Industrial injury which could be prevented by wearing mouth guard in boxers and head gear, the professional athletes reduce the sportive injury.

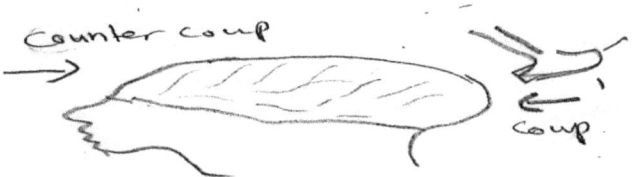

Figure28 direct (coup) and indirect injury (countercoup)

2.Indirect injury (countercoup injury)

1.Fall from height which is prevented by avoid living in the mounting, railing also avoid open plan windows in high buildings, follow legislations and rules and fear of litigation.

2.Crushing injury automobile accident e, aeroplane crash

Milling accident prevented by legislation and fear of litigations.

5.High velocity missile injury (war injury) it usually prevented by peace process.

6.Itatrogenic injury (the doctor is the cause of injury) it could occur by dentist doing fracture of the tooth during dental extraction by using uncontrollable force, it is commonly prevented by gaining operative skills and good training staff.

7.pathological injury that fracture of the facial bones by presence of cyst, tumour, osteomyelitis it could be prevented by early management of the patient.

<u>The Forces required to produce the fracture of the facial bone bones are as follows:</u>

The kinetic energy equal mass multiplied by velocity raise to force two.

K=mv2 (table4)

K=kinetic energy, m= mass. V=velocity

The bone fracture	The forces required
Nasal bone	30g
Zygomatic bone	50g
The mandibular angle	70g
The frontal bone	80g
The maxilla (midline)	100g
The mandible (midline)	100g
Supraorbital rim	200g

Table 4 Showing the different forces required to fracture the facial bones.

The prevalence of middle third fractures (tables5)

Fracture type		Prevalence
Zygomaticomaxillary complex (tripod fracture)		40%
Lefort	i	15%
Lefort	ii	!0 %
Lefort	iii	10%
Zygomatic arch		10%
Alveolar process of maxilla		5%
Smash fracture		5%
Others		5 %

Table5 Showing the prevalence of middle third fracture.

Chapter Three

The characteristic of middle third fracture

1.Fractures of numbers of bones (not isolated).

2.All bones are fragile in complex fashion.

3.Function as cushion against trauma to the brain.

4.Anatomical communicated complex pushed downward posteriorly (dish face)

5. The middle third complex protect the orifices (eye, nose, paranasal sinuses, brain, and cranial nerves).

6.Easily withstand the force of mastication and vertical forces from below but not superior or lateral or frontal forces.

7.If the middle third is removed from the skull the inclined pterygoid bone form bone 45degree with frontal bone resulting in premature gagging and anterior open bite and the soft palate push down to the pharynx.

8.The dorsum of the tongue can cause airway obstruction during trauma.

9.The gross disruption of maxilla lead to exposure of paranasal sinuses causing infection and the blood will occlude the nasal airway.

10. The communication of thin floor and medial wall of the orbit could lead to impairment of the orbital support.

11. The shear stress of ethmoidal region (cribriform plates) lead to CSF leakage (rhinorrhoea).

The classifications of middle third facial bone fractures

1.According to the type of fracture

1.Simple fracture it is linear fracture no external communication, no periosteal tear, in children is called the green stick fracture involving one cortical plate it is incomplete fracture.

2.Compound fracture it is bony fracture extended to external communication with skin or soft tissue or periodontal ligament and there is periosteal tear.

3.Comminuted fracture it is fracture of bone into small pieces.

4.Pathological fracture it is bone fracture due to presence of cyst, tumour, osteomyelitis that weakened the bone.

5.Iatrogenic fracture by dentist during tooth extraction or surgical procedure led to fracture of bone.

2.According to the site of fracture

A. Unilateral fracture

B. Bilateral fracture

Complex fracture it is compound fracture with damage to adjacent structures.

3.According to the aetiology of fracture

A. Civilian (no military) e.g., assault, fall, industrial injury, Road Traffic Accident (RTA,) sport, etc.

B. Non civilian fracture (military or war) e.g., gunshot, missile injuries. Etc.

The clinical feature of middle third fracture

1. Apparent trismus.
2. Lengthening of the midface.

3. Obtrusion of the airway by the soft palate resting on posterior dorsum of the tongue.
4. Dish face deformity.
5. Facial swelling
6. Bilateral circumorbital ecchymosis (panda face or raccoon eyes).
7. Abnormal mobility of the midface.
8. Pain over the nose or face.
9. Diplopia (double vision).
10. Anaesthesia or paraesthia in infraorbital nerve.

Chapter Four

The classification of middle third fractures

1.Dentoalveolar fracture.

2.Zygomatic complex fracture.

3.The nasal complex fracture.

4.Lefort i fracture.

5.Lefort ii fracture.

6.Lefort iii fracture.

Lefort fractures involving the occlusion.

1.Dentoalveolar fracture.

2.Lefort i fracture.

3.Lefort ii fracture.

4.Lefort iii fracture.

Lefort fractures not involving the occlusion.

  A.   In the central region
1.   Anterior nasal fracture.
2.   Lateral nasal fracture.

  B. Fractures of frontal process of maxilla

     1.Naso -ethmoidal fractures.
     2.Naso -ethomido- orbital fractures.
     3.Fronto- naso-ethmoido- orbital fractures.

The Lefort fractures

The weakest areas of midfacial complex when assaulted from a frontal direction at various levels coined by (Rene Lefort 1901)
Lefort i fracture it is located at level of the teeth.
Lefort ii fracture it is positioned above teeth level.
Lefort iii fracture it is at orbital level.

The classifications of Lefort fractures
1. According to fracture line (figure 29,30,31,32)
Lefort i low level fracture.
Lefort ii mid-level fracture.
Lefort iii high level fracture.

LeFort Fracture Classification

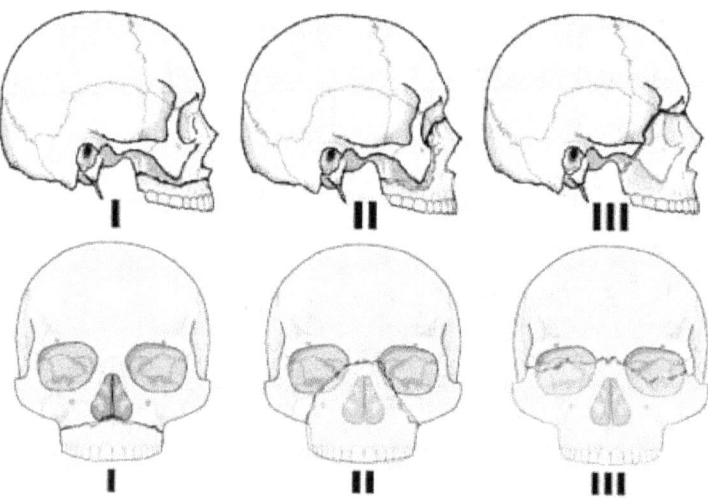

Figure 29

2.Accoring to fracture of the pterygoid lamina plate
 (Figure 29)

Lefort i in level lower third of pterygoid lamina fracture.
Lefort ii in level middle third of pterygoid lamina fracture.
Lefort iii in level of upper third of pterygoid lamina frac-
ture.

Lefort 1 fracture
   Has many names it called: -
1.Gurien fracture.
2.Horizontal fracture.
3.High dentoalveolar fracture because dentolvelar fracture is in the level of the teeth in upper jaw, so Lefort 1 is
above it.
4.low level fracture.
5.Floating fracture.
6.Ptregomaxillary disjunction.
7.Telescope fracture.
        The Lefort 1 fracture pass from and through these
structures
1.   lateral margin to anterior nasal aperture.
2.   Canine eminence.
3.   lateral wall of maxillary antrum.

4.Cross the zygomaticomaxillary sutures.

5.Below zygomatic buttress.

6.Lower third of pterygoid lamina.

Lefort 2 fracture

Has also different names

1.Subzygomatic fracture.

2.Mid-level fracture.

3.Pyramid fracture.

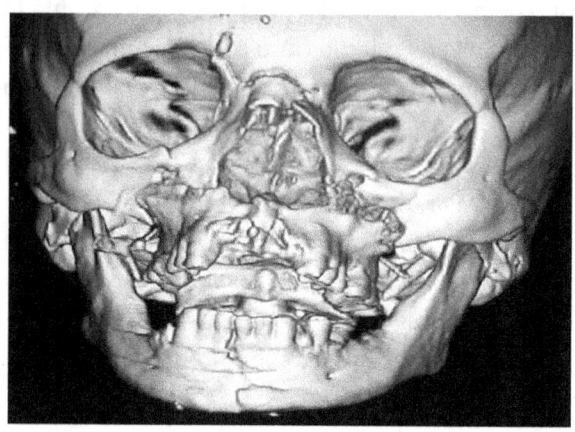

Figure30 showing 3deminsion (3D) CT facial bone Lefort 1,2 fracture.

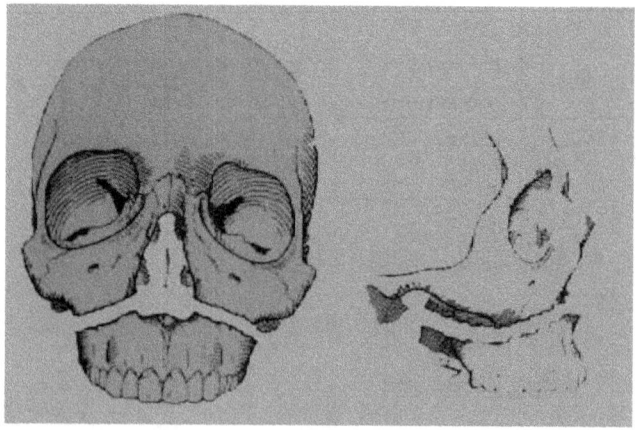

Figure 31 showing Lefort 1 fracture.

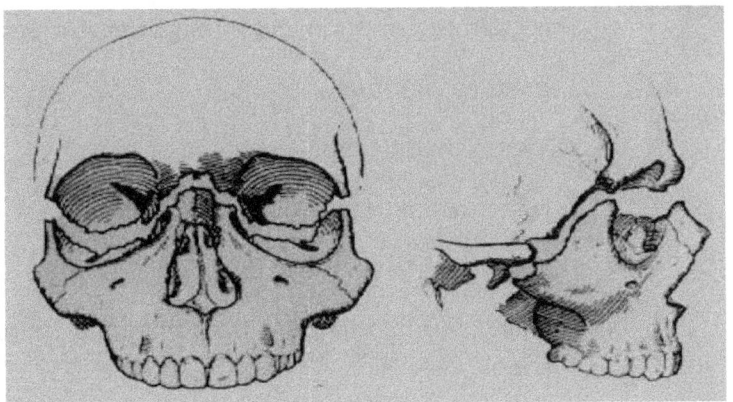

Figure 3 showing Lefort 2 fracture.

This fracture pass from and through these structures: -

1.frontal process of maxilla.

2.lateral wall of the orbit.

3.lacrimal bone.

4. infraorbital supervisors.

5.downward backward lateral wall of maxillary antrum.

6. cross zygomaticomaxillary suture.

7. Pterygoid lamina halfway.

Lefort 3 fracture

The different names of this type of fracture: -

1.suprazygomatic fracture.

2. High level fracture.

3. Transverse fracture.

4. Craniofacial disjunction.

This fracture pass from and through these structures

1.Frontonasal suture.

2.Below the optic supervisors.

3. Posterior limit of inferior orbital fissure.

Then it goes in one or two directions: -

1.Behind the maxilla then fract the upper third of the Pterygoid lamina.

2.or fract the frontozygomatic suture and the zygomatic arch.

There are two pillars in the maxillary skeleton, (Figure 33)

A. The horizontal pillars.
B. The vertical pillars
A. The horizontal pillars of the maxillary Skelton are: -
    1.the superior pillars are the supraorbital rim.
    2. the middle pillars are the infraorbital rim.
    3. the inferior pillars are the alveolar process.

B.   The vertical pillars of the maxillary Skelton are: -
    1.The anterior pillars are canine pillars
    2.The middle pillars are zygomatic pillars
    3.The posterior pillars are the pterygoid pillars.

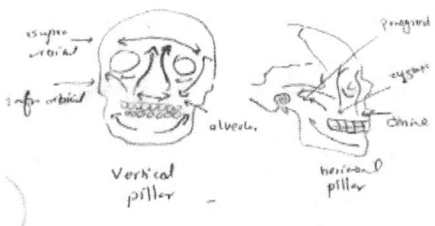

Figure 33 vertical and horizontal pillars of maxillary skeleton

The hot points in middle third fracture

1. The frontonasal suture fracture associated with Lefort 2 fracture.
2. The frontozygomatic suture fracture associated with Lefort 3 fracture and zygomatic bone fracture.
3. The pterygoid plate fracture of sphenoid bone associated with Lefort 1 or 2 or 3

According to the level of pterygoid plate fracture, if the upper part (Lefort 1) the middle part (lefort2), lower part fracture of pterygoid plate of sphenoid (lefor3) fracture.

The classification of middle third fractures

A. According to zygomatic bone relation

1. Subzyomatic bone fracture (both lefort1 and Lefort 2).
2. Supra zygomatic bone fracture (Lefort 3)

A. According to the direction of fracture line

1.The horizontal fracture (Lefort 1)
2. The pyramidal fracture (lefort2)
3. The transverse fracture (lefort3).

The clinical feature of Lefort 1 fracture

1. Oedema of upper jaw and swelling.
2. Bilateral epistaxis (bleeding from the nose).
3. Ecchymosis (redness) of the buccal mucosa.
4. Occlusal disturbance.
5. Pain while speaking and moving of the jaw.
6. Cracked cup or pot sound during teeth percussion.
7.Upward displacement of the maxillary teeth (telescope fracture)
8.Mobility of the teeth bearing segment.

The clinical features of Lefort 2) fracture

1. Step deformity of infraorbital region.
2. Anaesthesia or paraesthesia of the cheek.
3. Oedema in the middle part of the face.
4. Movement of the maxilla as one segment with the nasal bone.

The clinical features of Lefort 3 fracture

1.Enopthalmos

2.Diplopia (double vision)

3.Hooding of the eye (ptosis like read).
3. Step deformity in frontozygomatic suture.
4. Fracture of zygomatic arch.
5. Panda face
6. Mobility of all skeletons as one block.
7. Palatal split.
8. Dish face.
9. Tele canthus (increase interpupillary distance more than 35 mm.

The clinical feature of Lefort 2,3 together

Inspection: -

1.Oedema of the face.

2. Circumorbital ecchymosis of the eye.

3.Subconjuctival haemorrhage

4.Lenghenig of the face.

5. Rhinorrhoea (CSF leakage through the nose).

6. Epitasis (bleeding per nose).

7.Nasal flatness or nasal deformity.

8.Retroposition of the maxilla and gagging of the occlusion.

9. Hematoma and bruising of the palate (Guerin sign) it occurs due to the palatal split.

Palpation

1.step deformity in the orbital rim.

2.crack pot sound in the maxillary teeth.

3. tenderness in fracture line area.

The management of the middle third fracture

Preliminary treatment

A, B, C, D, E.

Clerking (patient history).

Clinical examination

inspection, palpation, percussion.

1.Intraoral examination.

2.Extra oral examination.

3.Investigations.

4.Diagnosis.

5.Treatment planning

6. Definitive treatment

Preliminary treatment

A, B, C, D, E.

A-Airway and cervical spine control

B- Breathing

C. Circulation

D– Disability

E. Exposure and environmental control

Airway

Ask the patient if he is all, right?

The maintenance of the airway depends on the following.

1.   Absence of any anatomical or mechanical barrier.
2.   Preservation of laryngeal reflex.
3.   Existence of pulmonary ventilation.
4.   The integrity of the respiratory centre.

     The treatment is to maintain the patent airway.

     To preserve the level of consciousness.

The Position of the patient

The head position in unconscious patient (the coma position).

Chin lift, jaw thrust.

Suction or manual removal of foreign body in the mouth (removal of blood clot, vomitus, bone, teeth).

Endotracheal intubation

Mouth to moth breathing or mouth to nose breathing especially in children or infant.

Tracheostomy

Anterior traction of the tongue

Restoration of soft palate position

Oro or nasopharyngeal airway

Nasotracheal intubation should be avoided in the patient with midface trauma to prevent passage of the tube through the fractured cribriform plate into the brain.

The surgical management of the airway

(Tracheostomy).

Indications of tracheostomy

1.Lack of tongue control.
2.Gross retro position of middle third fracture of facial skeleton.
3.Potential oedema of pharynx and glottis.
4.Uncontrol of oropharyngeal bleeding.
5.Inadequate pulmonary and CNS depression.

Breathing

Ventilation should be assessed.
Injury compromise ventilation.
Tension pneumothorax.
Cardiac tamponade.
Massive hemopneumothorax.
Rupture diaphragm.

Clinical examination
Deviated trachea.
Absence of breath sound.
Dullness of percussion.
Muffled heart sound.
Radiological check

Loss of lung marking.
Deviated trachea.
Raised hemidiaphragm.
Fluid level.
Treatment

Chest drainage – chest tube placed in 4 intercostal space anterior to mid axillary line.
Cardiac tamponade is treated by decompensation of pericardium with needle guided by ECG.

Give oxygen supplement.
Circulation (bleeding)

the management of bleeding could be treated as follows: -
1.Fluid replacement
2.Put cannula
3.Crystaloid solution as ringer lactate which correct hypovo-lemic shock which occur after loss of 40% of blood.
4. The circulation volume of adult is 7% of body weight is five litres in 70kg pt and 80-90 ml/kg in the child.
5.blood sample take 3cc of blood and do cross matching and Hb level.
6. Vital signs monitoring blood pressure (BP) =120-150 /80-95, Temperature 37 degree centigrade (98,4F), respiratory rate 12-18 breath/minute. (B/M}
Pulse 72 to 100 (B/M) and 120 in school child and 140 in pre-school child and 160 in infant (less than 2 years)
7.Blood transfusion.
8.Posterior nasal pack in case of bleeding from posterior na-sal aperture.
Clinical examination

1.Tachycardia.
2.Hypotension.
3.Narrow pulse pressure.
4.Tachypnoea.
5.Delayed capillary return.
6.Falling of urinary output (UOP) normally it is 50ml per hour in adult 1m/kg in 1 year child and 2ml/kg in child below 1 year.
7.Deterioration of mental status.
Disability

Transportation of the patient

Put the patient in coma position in lateral position and supine position in case of cervical collar fracture and support cervical spine (Figure 10).

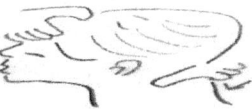

Figure 34 neck support in case of cervical region

Neurological deficit

Check the transport of the patient without movement of vertebral column in case of cervical fracture.
10% of the unconscious patient sustain road traffic accident of the patient have a chance of cervical spine injury (Figure34).

Management of cervical injury

Semi- rigid cervical collar, spine board, bolstering device, if the patient is unconscious send him for neurosurgeon.
Examination of pupil
Indications
1. Trauma to the brain.
2. Optic tract trauma
3. Progess of the patient after the trauma.
Papilledema, vomiting, neurological deficit and amentia, dilation of and fixation of pupil. Irritation due to cerebral ischemia or hypoxia are sinister sign of the brain injury.
Check the Glasco Coma Scale (GCS) that.
1. Asertain the level of consciousness
2. it ascertain eye, motor, verbal response.
Which it is 15 Scales from 3 to 15 scores
Eye response are 4 scores.

Verbal response are 5 scores.

Motor response are 6 scores.

Eye opening

Are 4 scores.

1 is none.

4 is spontaneous eye opening.

Spontaneous eye opening to pain is score 2, pinch the patient or press him he will open his eyes.

Spontaneous eye opening to speech is score 3 ask the patient to open his eyes.

The verbal response

The verbal response are 5 scores.

1 is none or no response.

5 the pt is fully oriented.

Sound, word, speech(conversation) is (2,3,4) scores, respectively.

2 is incomprehensive sound.

3 is inappropriate word.

4 is confused conversion.

Motor response

Motor response or movement are 6 scores.

1 is none.

6 is obey the order.

2 is extension of the hand and leg away from the body. (Decorticated patient), (Figure35).

3 is abnormal flexion of the hand and leg collected to the body. (Figure35).

(Decerebrated patient).

4 is withdraw if you pinch him.

5 is localized the pain, ask the patient where the site of pain is after you pinch him.

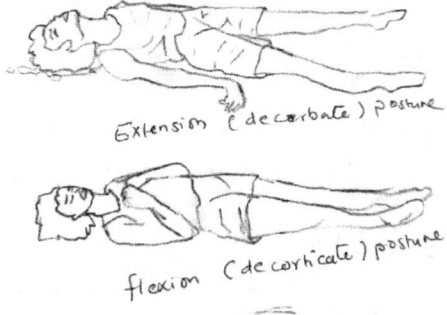

Figure 35 decerebrate and decorticate posture.

AVPU Scale

AVPU are 4 points scales. Which is quicker scale in comparison to GCS.

A-Awake

V-Verbal stimulus

P-Painful stimulus

U-Unconscious patient.

The injury to the middle cranial fossa

In case of to the middle cranial fossa injury the patient complains

1.Rgurgitation.

2.Abscence of gag reflex

3.Weakness of the voice.

Cerebrospinal fluid (CSF), (Table3)

Cerebrospinal fluid (CSF) is a clear, colorless body fluid found within the tissue that surrounds the brain and spinal cord of all vertebrates.

CSF is produced by specialised ependymal cells in the choroid plexus of the ventricles of the brain, and absorbed in the arachnoid granulations. There is about 125 mL of CSF at any one time, and about 500 mL is generated every day. CSF acts as a shock absorber, cushion or buffer, providing basic mechanical and immunological protection to the brain inside the skull. CSF also serves a vital function in the cerebral autoregulation of cerebral blood flow.

CSF produce by choroids plexus; the fluid surrounds the brain and the spinal cord.

In the brain. orbital frontal bone, cribriform plate of ethmoidal bone in Lefort 3 fracture and Lefort 2 and Naso ethomido orbital fracture.

1.checking of protein, glucose level of CSF.

2.Testing for beta2 transferrin is substance found only in CSF.

Meningitis is fatal complication of CSF leakage through the nose (rhino rhea) or CSF leakage through the ear (otorrhea), so the lumber drainage (lumber puncture) is the treatment of choice.

Constituent	CSF	Serum	Nasal secretion
Osmolarity	295 mOsm/L	295 mOsm/L	277 mOsm/L
Glucose	58-900mg/100ml	80-120mg/100mL	14-32mg/100mL
Albumin	50-75%	55%	57%
Total protein	5-45mg/dL	6.0-8.4mg/dL	335-636mg/dL
B2- transferrin	15% of total Transferrin	0%	0%

Table 6 showing the different between the CSF, serum, nasal secretion.

We could use cotton gauze to differentiate the nasal secretion from CSF which appear as two halo the blood in the centre.

In CT brain CSF appearance as tram line (figure36)

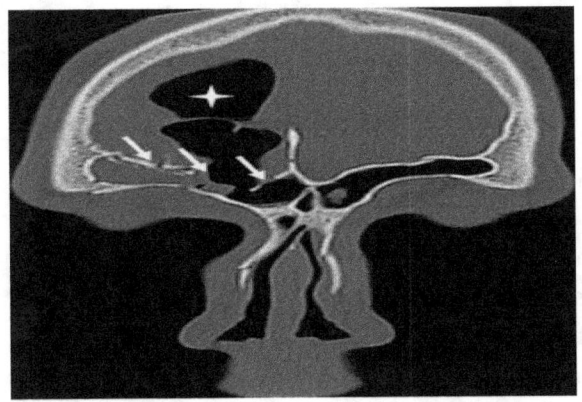

Figure36 tram track appearance CSF leakage

Exposure and environmental control
To discover other injuries

Chest, abdominal, limbs and pelvis injuries.
Ask the patient to take his close off to see the other fractures and put him in suitable temperature and environment.
Intraperitoneal bleeding diagnosis by

Frank blood on aspiration.
More than 1000 leukocytes.
More than 500 erythrocytes.
Bowel content.
Urine.
Loss of blood in limb trauma
Tibia fracture 1.5units.
Fibula fracture 1.5 units.
Femur is 3 units.
Pelvis is 3 units of blood loss.

History

Ask the patient if he is All right?

The date and time of trauma?

How the trauma occurs? The mode and direction of trauma?

The object by which trauma occur sharp or blunt?

If the patient loss his conscious?

If the patient has amentia?

Is it retrograde amentia is failure to remember up to the time of injury?

Anterograde amentia is loss of memory following trauma.

If the bleeding occurs from the nose or nose, mouth, or ear?

If rhino rhea or otorrhea had occur?

If the patient had any other type of trauma in the body?

If the patient seen by neurosurgeon or any other department -if the answer is yes

The time and duration of admission?

The medication taken during admission period.

If any medication taken prior to accident especially anticoagulant, steroids, insulin, narcotics analgesics?

The patient is medically fit or not but if the answer is no. what is other type of the disease the patient has?

If the patient control or not?

If the patient had followed up with another physician?

If the patient

If excessive amount of blood had been lost?

If any complication had been occurring during the time of admission?

If the patient had any blood transfusion?

If the patient had any legal consent?

If the patient had been referred?

If the patient finished his treatment?

Radiological examination

Occipitomental view or sinus view.

CT facial bone 2 or 3 dimensions (2D,3D).

Lateral skull view for fracture nasal bone.

Submentovertex vertex view to see the zygomatic arch fracture or base of skull fracture.

Periapical and occlusal views for dentoalveolar fracture.

MRI for soft tissues

PA skull view if there is associated bone fracture.

OPG X-ray to see if there is associated fracture mandible.

Investigations

Complete blood picture and serum and electrolytes.

CT facial bone MRI head and neck.

Other x-rays e.g., Hand. leg if associated with other types of fractures.

C-spine.

Chest x-rays.

ECG.

The physician should check the general patient condition.

Physician report.

Patient for hospital admission for document and file.

Preoperative preparation

Patient bath, nasogastric tube, shaving and oral hygiene by brushing.

Premedication's e.g., Anxiolytic drugs, antibiotics,

Operative consent.

Definitive treatment
Principle of middle third definitive treatment

1.loss of infection.

2.Reduction.

3.Immobilization.

4.Rehabilitaton.

The intermaxillary fixation prevent the anterior posterior movement in Lefort fracture.

Suspension prevents lateral movement for Lefort fracture.
Plating system may not need intermaxillary fixation.

Circular facial Treatment

Teeth and occlusion are the key to reconstruction and provide the foundation upon which other facial structures are built.
1. From outside to inside.
2. Bone before mucosa.
3. 3.lower before upper jaw fixation.
   Surgical treatment planning
   Timing of surgical procedure
   Emergency treatment is resuscitating the patient.
   Stabilization of the mobile fracture to maintain airway need for tracheostomy.
   Arrest haemorrhage and transfuse blood if necessary.
   Control of soft tissues lacerations
   Control of pain
   Control of infection
   Timing of surgical procedure
   Within 2-4 hours
   Repair deep lacerations

Impression of the teeth.

Treat the less severe maxillary fracture if no other injuries.

Definitive treatment between the 2-7 days.

Improve the medical condition of the patient.

Careful clinical assessment and planning

Reduction of soft tissue and oedema and swelling.

Planning of incision

The Skeletal incision in middle third fracture

1. Supraorbital eyebrow incision.
2. Sub ciliary incision.
3. Median lower eyelid incision
4. Infraorbital incision transconjunctival incision
5. Transconjunctival incision
6. Zygomatic arch incision.
7. Transverse nasal incision.
8. Vertical nasal incision.
9. Medial orbital incision.
10. Open sky incision.
11. Unitemporal (unicronal) incision.
12. Bi temporal (bicronal) incision.

The stages of surgical procedure of multiple facial fractures

Dentoalveolar fracture

The extraction of the teeth beyond repair

Reduction and fixation of dentoalveolar fractures

Reduction of the mandibular fracture to guide for correct position of the maxilla.

The zygomatic bone fractures the zygoma should be elevated to allow greater disimpaction and reduction.

The management of middle third fractures and methods of reduction and immobilization

1.reduction

A. Open reduction means open the area of fracture surgically.

A-Internal

ionone rigid Fixation

Close reduction

Immobilization (intermaxillary fixation IMF)

Skeletal fixation which could be divided into

Suspension wiring and intermedullary pins.

Trans fixation K Wire.

Trans facial.

Zygomatic septal

Transossus wiring.

ii) Rigid fixation.

Adaptive plate

Mono-cortical screws

A – external fixation

External pin fixation via

Halo frame.

Plaster of Paris.

Box frame.

B-Internal

I non rigid

Suspension wiring (Figure37)

1. Pyriform aperture suspension (Adam wire).
2. Infraorbital suspension.

3. Circum zygomatic suspension.
4. Frontal suspension (Kufner).
5. Circumplatal suspension.
6. Cranial suspension (Thoma).

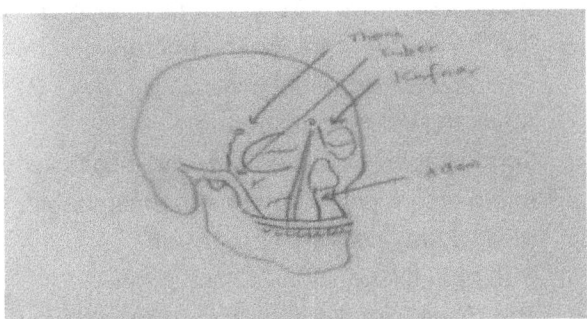

Figure 37 showing wire suspension in middle third facial injury.

Transossus wiring internal fixation.

1. Direct osteosynthesis
2. Transossus wiring.
3. high level frontozygomatic (frontonasal).
4. Mid-level (orbital rim, zygomatic buttress)
5. Low level (midpalatal)
   ii.Rigid
   adaptational plate
   compressive plate or lag screw
   support
   antral pack.
   antral balloon.
   Principles of plating mid face
   Must restore the supporting pillars up to the masticatory forces.
   Miniplates must lie in the longitudinal direction of these pillars.

Mini cortical, orbit, nasoethmoidal areas.

Compression plates, sometimes used in the mandible.

Wire suspension

Adam 1942 wire suspension to reduce and suspend mobile fragment above the fracture line by mean of 0.5 mm stainless steel wire.

Advantage of wire suspension

Comfortable, well tolerated, and inconspicuous.

Rapid technique, accurate and dependable.

Disadvantage of wire suspension

Non rigid fixation

The suspension wires may excrete backward and upward pull which may lead to replase of reduced maxilla.

It requires intermaxillary fixation (IMF).

External skeletal fixation

Involve the use of external rods and universal joints which links the cranium above the fracture line to the mandible or maxilla via extension wire rigidly attach to the teeth.

Hallo frame.

Levant frame.

Box frame.

The complications of the maxillary fracture

Preoperative complications

Airway displacement of the maxilla displaced it causes the soft palate to rest on dorsum tongue surface.

Epistaxis is nasal bleeding from the maxillary arteries.

Inhalation of the tooth fragment.

Post operative complications.

Excessive bleeding may need blood transfusion.

Infection

Wound dehiscence

Emphysema.

Meningitis due to CSF leakage.

Malocclusion.

Facial scaring.

Rehabilitation

Facial scar revision

Dental rehabilitation

Periodontal rehabilitation

Post traumatic facial deformity correction.

Social and psychiatric report and rehabilitation

Posture put the patient in supine position in conscious patient and lateral position in comatose patient.

Give sedation.

Prevention of infection 'oral hygiene.

Feeding and nutrition.

Mainting the occlusion.

Viability of teeth damage by (pulp test).

Paraesthesia of lower jaw.

Gingivitis.

Control of primary complications

Infection

Nerve damage

Displacement of the teeth

Present of foreign body

Pulpitis.

Periodontal condition and gingiva.

Drug reaction.

Control of late complications

Mal union.

Non-union.

Derangement of TMJ.

Sequestration of the bone.

Traumatic myositis ossificans. Scars

Chapter Five

Zygomatic complex fracture Figure (38,39)

Zygoma is prominent buttress of the cheek located in the lateral portion of the middle third of facial skeleton.
The zygomatic bone has common 2nd injury after the nose.
Because the nose is more prominent than zygoma
It is a dense bone has 4-points structures or tripod fracture.
It called malar or zygoma.

Boundaries of the zygomatic complex fracture

Superiorly attached to the frontal bone.
Inferiorly there is buccal sulcus.
Laterally attached to the temporal bone.
Sutures attachments
1.The zygomaticofacial suture.
2.Tthe zygomatico temporal suture.
3.The frontozygomatic suture.
4. the zygomatico sphenoid suture.

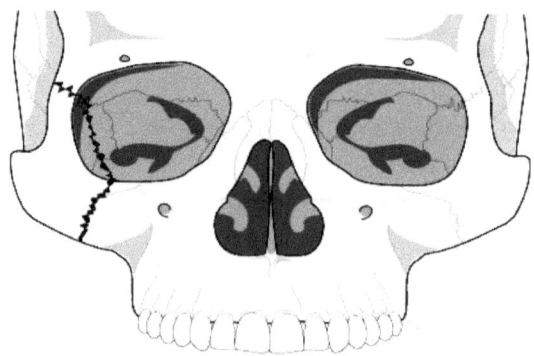

Figure38 fracture zygoma front view

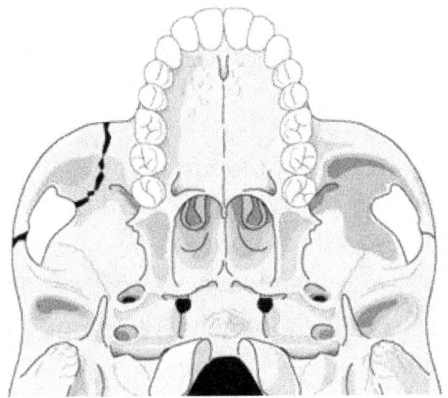

Figure 39 fracture zygoma above view

The function of the zygoma

The vertical and horizontal pillars
1.Protection of the eye globe.
2.Give the origin of masseter muscle.
3.Transmit part of the masticatory force to the brain.
The articulation of the zygoma with the adjacent craniofacial structures

The zygomatico frontal suture.
The infraorbital rim.
The zygomaticomaxillary buttress.
The zygomatic arch.
The zygomatico sphenoid suture.

Figure 13 showing the vertical and horizontal buttress.

<u>The complications of untreated</u> <u>zygomatic complex fracture</u>
Flat cheek.
Enophthalmos.
Alter pupil level (hypo or hyper Globus).
Infraorbital paraesthesia.
Diplopia (double vision).
Impaired mandibular movement (change of occlusion).
<u>The classification of zygomatic bone fracture (Figure 40)</u>

1.Minimal or no displacement.
2.Inward downward displacement.
3.Inward and posterior displacement.
4. Comminuted complex fracture.

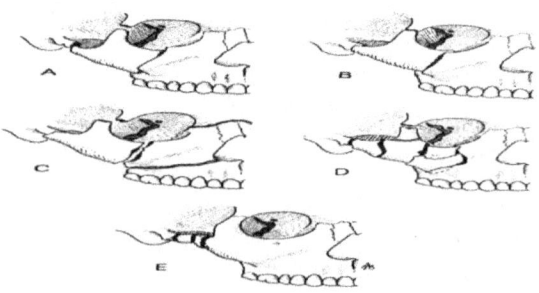

Figure 40 showing classification of zygomatic bone fracture.

<u>The classification of the zygomatic arch fracture</u>

1.Minimal or no displacement.

2.V – shaped inward displacement.

3.v- shaped outward displacement.

4.Comminuted zygomatic arch fracture.

The clinical feature of zygomatic bone fracture

The Face

Moon face

The orbital rim

Tenderness over orbital rim

Step deformity

The occlusion

Gagging of the occlusion

Closed position it is type of fracture during sudden opening of the mouth.

Open position it is type of fracture that occur during sudden closure of the mouth.

Limitation of the mandibular movement.

The nerve

Anaesthesia is complete loss of sensation.

Paraesthesia is partial loss of sensation.

Neurotmesis is complete injury of the nerve.

Neuropraxia is partial injury of the nerve.

Extraoral examination

The eyes

Circumorbital ecchymosis.

Subconjunctival haemorrhage.

Limitation of ocular movement.

Diplopia.

Strabismus

Enophthalmos (inside sinking of the eye)

The mouth opening.

Limitation of lateral excursion of mandible toward inured side.

Limitation of opening and closing of the mandible.

The nose

Unliteral epitaxies (bleeding per nose).

The extraoral examination

On palpation

The cheek

Oedema of the cheek

Flattening of the zygoma.

The orbit

Notching in the lower rim of the orbit in the region of fronto-zygomatic region at lateral side of the orbit.

The nerve

Anaesthesia or paraesthesia of the cheek.

Intraoral examination

Inspection

Buccal region

Ecchymosis in the upper buccal sulcus in the zygomatic buttress.

Occlusion

Gagging of the occlusion in the molar region in the injured side.

On palpation

Buccal region

Tenderness in the upper buccal sulcus in the zygomatic buttress.

Anaesthesia in the upper gum

The cheek

Flatting and swelling of the cheek

Viewing the patient

Two views of the patient

1.viewing from above (bird view), (Figure 18)

2. viewing the zygoma from below. To compare the right and left cheek.

Haemorrhage of the orbit (Figure 41)

Anterior to the orbital septum

Subperiosteal haematoma

Haemorrhage within the oscular muscle cone (intraconal haemorrhage).

Intracranial haemorrhage could spread to the orbit to superior orbital fissure and optic foramen,

The unlimited eye ecchymosis indicated the zygomatic bone fracture.

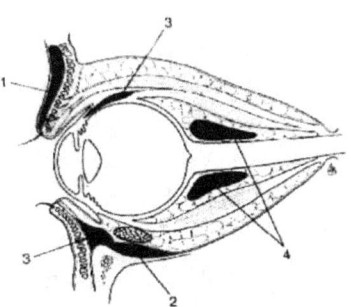

The locations of haemorrhage in the orbital area which can occur after fracture or contusion. 1, Lid ecchymosis. 2, Subperiosteal haematoma. 3, Haemorrhage posterior to the orbital septum including subconjunctival haemorrhage. 4, Haemorrhage within the muscle cone.

Figure 41showing orbital haemorrhage.

the clinical feature of orbital injury in the zygomatic bone fracture

periorbital haematoma.

limitation of ocular movement

subconjunctival haemorrhage

diplopia

enophthalmos

lowering of the pupil level

tele canthus (hypertelorism) it is increase of interpupillary distance.

The eyeball suspended by suspensory lock wood ligament which run from the Whinnall.

Tubercle which located just below the zygomaticofrontal suture to the inner wall of the orbital rim .so the fracture above the zygomaticofrontal suture it led to diplopia (double vision).

But the fracture below the zygomaticofrontal suture did not change the ocular level.

The causes of diplopia are: -
1. The fracture above the Whinnall tubercle
2. Haematoma or oedema of extraocular muscle
3. Fibrosis of the ocular muscle.

The types of diplopia

Mononuclear diplopia it occurs in one eye ask the pt to close one eye during the diplopia test, this type is more serious because it indicates true eye injury.

The binocular diplopia- occurs in both eyes, the form of diplopia is not serious may be due to

Oedema or hematoma in both eyes.

Hess chart (nine gauze test)

This test is asking the patient to see the doctor finger 6 inches away in different 8 direction of encompass and to the centre.

Aim of treatment of the zygomatic bone fracture

1.To restore the normal contour of the face.

2.To re-establish the skeletal protection of the eye globe.

3.To correct the ocular changes

4.To prevent the interference with range of movement of the mandible.

Classification of zygomatic bone fracture

Type A: Incomplete low-energy fracture with fracture of only one zygomatic pillar

Type B: Complete mono-fragment fracture with fracture and displacement along all four articulations

Type C: Multi-fragmented, Comminuted fractures of the zygomatic body.

The management of fracture zygoma
The surgical planning of different incisions
Extraoral and Orbital incision

Gilles approach

Lateral brow incision

Medical canthus incision

Sub ciliary incision.

Midtarsal incision.

Orbital rim incision.

Intraoral incisions

Vestibular incision.

Semilunar incision.

Submarginal incision.

Gingival marginal incision.

Radiology

CT facial bone (axial, coronal ,3D) with high resolution thin cuts 0.6 mm to 1mm (figures19.21,22)

The surgical procedures of the zygomatic bone fracture
1. The external zygomatic hook
2. The Gilles temporal approach by row zygomatic elevator
3. Bristow elevator.

Gilles approach 1927 (Figure 42)

Incision in the temporal fascia

The bristo elevator is passed down to the zygomatic arch between the temporal fascia and temporalis muscles.

Elevation of the zygomatic bone or arch in correct anatomical position, we hear the sound click the two bones coming together.

Suture the fascia with resorbable Suture (vicryl or catgut)
Suture of the skin with non-resorbable suture (proline).

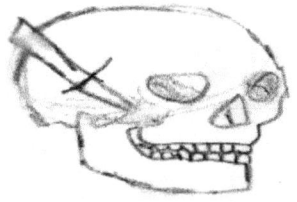

Figure 42 showing Gilles approach.

Keen approach intraoral upper buccal vestibular incision
By Internal zygomatic hook.
Dingman zygomaticofrontal incision by applying transossus wiring of zygomaticofrontal suture and infraorbital rim.
Pin fixation from zygomatic bone to supraorbital rim.
plating system by open reduction and internal fixation (ORIF) of zygomatic bone. (Figure 43)
There is risk of facial nerve injury.

Supporting the orbital rim by nasal pack or by antral balloon.

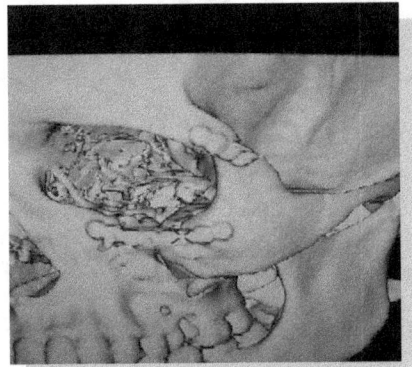

Figure 43 ORIF in left zygoma

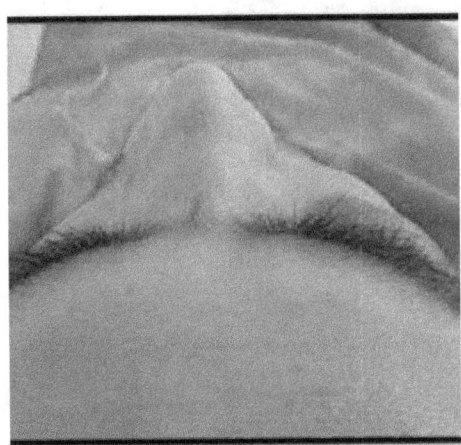

Figure 44 bird view

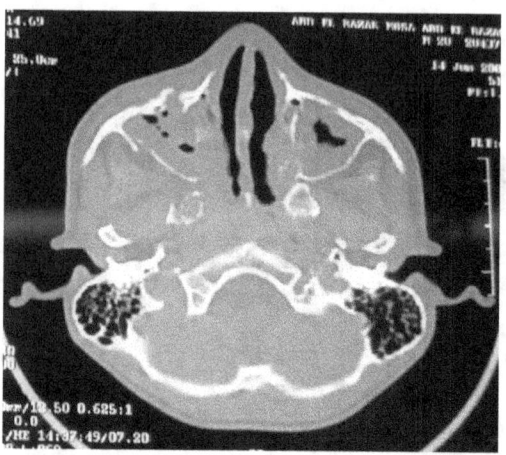

Figure 45 showing CT facial bone showing axial view zygomatic bone fracture.

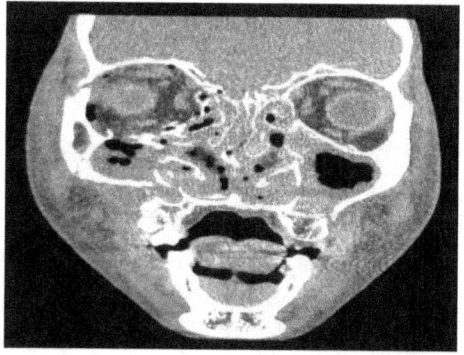

Figure 46 showing CT facial bone showing coronal view zygomatic bone fracture.

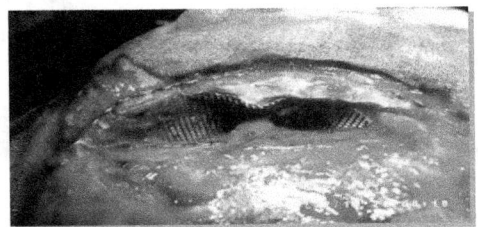

Figure 47 bicronal incision and orbital reconstruction by titanium mesh.

Fracture of zygomatic arch

The zygomatic arch fracture may be isolated fracture it contains of zygoma, maxilla and squamous temporal bone or associated with the zygomatic buttress.

The limitation of lateral excursion is the common feature of zygomatic arch fracture to impinge of the zygomatic arch with coronoid process it is immediate complication of zygomatic bone fracture.

The radiological examination

Submentovertex view to see the zygomatic arch fracture (Figure29)

The clinical feature of the zygomatic arch fracture

1.pain.

2.proptosis (the eyeball pushed forward) it is protrusion of eyeball

Note the difference between the proptosis and exophthalmos.

Proptosis is terminology used in trauma and exophthalmos is case of pathology like hyperparathyroidism, but the two terminology has the same meaning.

3.pupil dilatation.

4.opthalmoplegia.

5.low visual acuity.

Blowout fracture (Figure 46,48.49)

The orbit is composed of seven bones. The floor is formed by the sphenoid bone, the orbital process of the palatine bone, and the orbital process of the maxillary bone. The lateral wall is formed by the greater wing of the sphenoid bone posteriorly and the zygomatic and frontal bones anteriorly. The medial wall is made of the lesser wing of the sphenoid, the ethmoid bone, the lacrimal bone, and the frontal process of the maxilla. The roof of the orbit is composed of the frontal and sphenoid bones.

By age 5 years, orbital growth is 85% complete, and it is finalized between 7 years of age and puberty. An adult orbit has an average volume of 30 cc with the globe volume being around 7 cc. The height of the orbit is on average around 35 mm, whereas the width is approximately 40 mm as measured at the rims. The child's orbit is rounder, but with age the width increases. From the medial orbital rim to the apex measures approximately 45 mm in length

Hyphema is the layering of blood in the anterior chamber of the globe, usually from the tearing of blood vessels at the root of the iris. It may present with pain, blurred vision, and photophobia.

Inferior orbital fissure: This is located about 1 cm posterior to the inferolateral oribital rim.

It connects the pterygopalatine fossa with the floor of the orbit. Contents include sensory nerves.

V2 (infraorbital and zygomatic nerves), inferior ophthalmic vein and branches to pterygoid plexus,

and parasympathetic branches of the pterygopalatine ganglion. Contents of this fissure are usually.

reflected for proper inferior orbital floor exposure during surgery.

• Superior orbital fissure: This is located near the apex of the orbit. It serves as a conduit for cranial.

nerves III, IV, and VI and the first division of cranial nerve V (ophthalmic branch). Additionally, it

contains the superior ophthalmic vein and anastomosis of recurrent lacrimal and middle meningeal.

arteries. Fractures affecting this structure can lead to ophthalmoplegia, upper eyelid ptosis, pupillary.

dilatation, and forehead anesthesia, also known as superior orbital fissure syndrome.

• Optic canal: This is located at the apex of the orbit, just medial to the superior orbital fissure. It is about.

5 mm wide and less than 1 cm long.

Winnall's tubercle: (Figure 47) is located on the lateral orbital wall just below the frontozygomatic suture.

about 1 cm posterior to the lateral rim

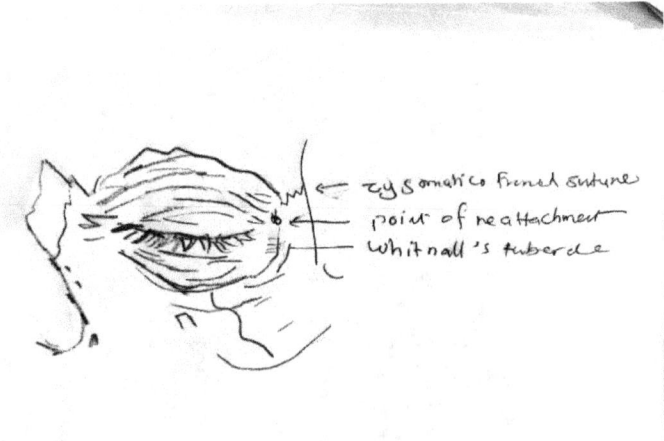

Figure 47 Whinnall tubercle

The orbit is pyramidal in shape, the apex is located at the optic foramen, the orbital floor is made of maxillary bone which is a part of zygomatic bone.

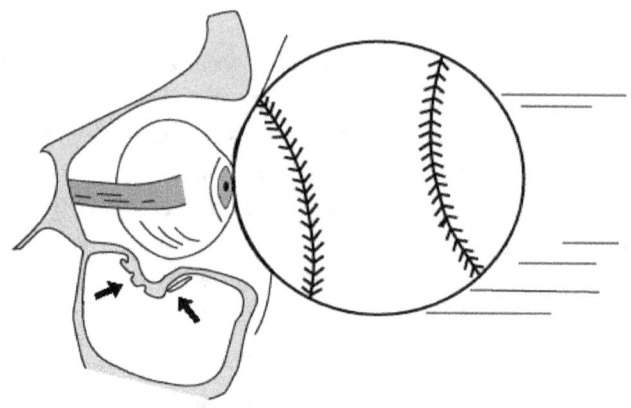

Figure 48 viewing the mechanism of bow out fracture direct orbital injury.

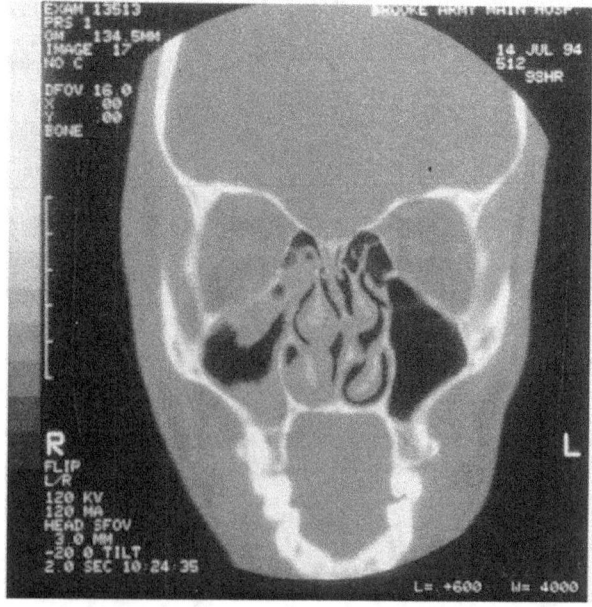

Figure 49 CT facial bone coronal view showing right orbit blow out fracture.

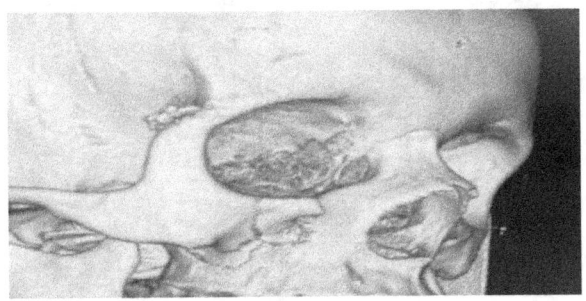

Figure 50 viewing zygomatic bone fracture and orbital rim fracture frontal view.

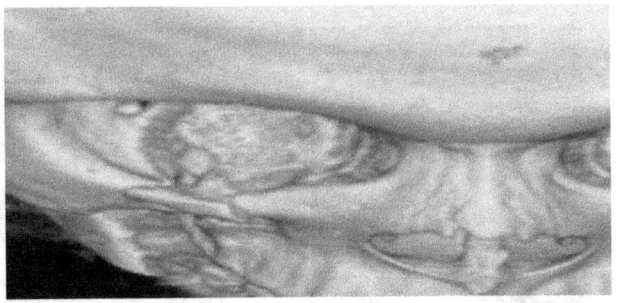

Figure51 CT facial bone showing zygomatic bone fracture and orbital rim fracture.

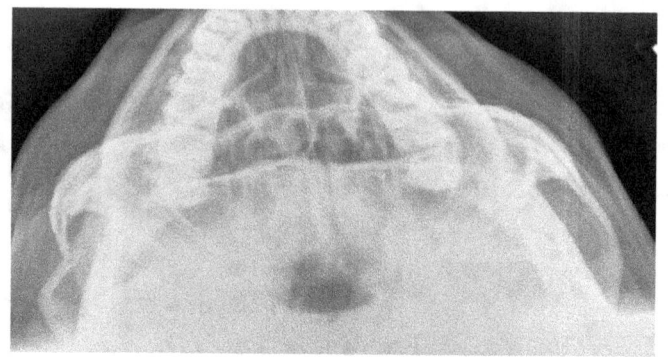

Figure 52 Submentovertex view showing right zygomatic arch fracture.

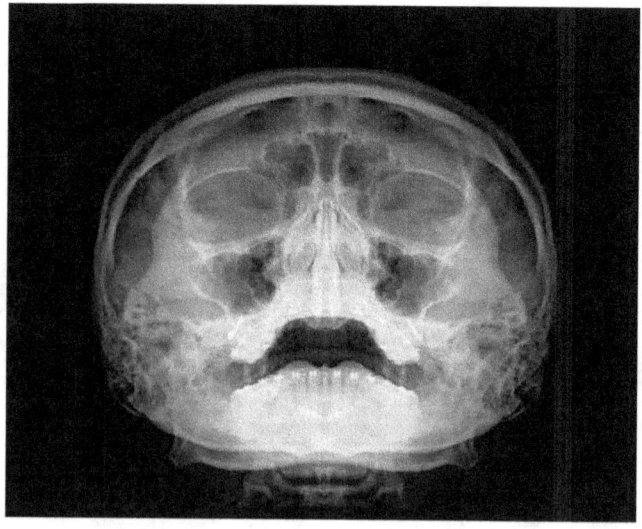

Figure 53 water view for maxillary sinus

The orbit is bounded laterally by the inferior orbital fissure and medially by the lacrimal bone, posteriorly it bounded by the orbital process of the palatine bone and part of ethmoidal bone.

The blow out fracture mechanism

Direct trauma to the orbit by ball push the orbit the floor and fracture it.

Indirect trauma to zygoma lead to blow out fracture.

The eyeball form only 1/3 of the orbital volume and the posterior 2/3 formed by fat and connective tissue and blood vessels, below the floor of the orbit is maxillary sinus (sinus of Highmore) the orbital floor forms the roof of the maxillary antrum (Figure53).

In cause of orbital trauma, the herniation of the orbit and his content into the maxillary sinus it called blow out fracture, but the periosteum may be attached to it (trap door appearance or hanging tear drop appearance).

The inferior oblique muscle and the inferior rectus muscle are attached to one sheath that affected with herniation of the orbital fat will lead to enophthalmos.

The clinical feature of blow out fracture.

Enophthalmos.

Disequilibrium of the orbital volume and contents.

Enlarged orbital volume.

Less orbital contents.

The investigations of blow out fracture.

Forced duct test suture the pulling of the inferior rectus and inferior oblique muscles by forceps or suture upward to assess the function in anaesthetize patient.

Occipitomental view to Hang drop or trap door appearance with maxillary sinus opacity or obliteration.

The treatment of blow out fracture.

Bone graft (Figure 32) in the lower orbital rim or sialastic material to prevent the sinking of the eye into the maxillary antrum or bone graft from the anterior antral wall or from ilia crest or titanium mesh for orbital reconstruction to support the globe of the eye (Figure 31).

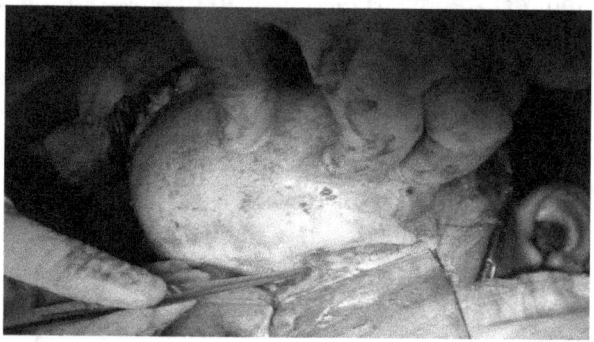

Figure 54 bicronal flap and ORIF for frontozygomatic suture

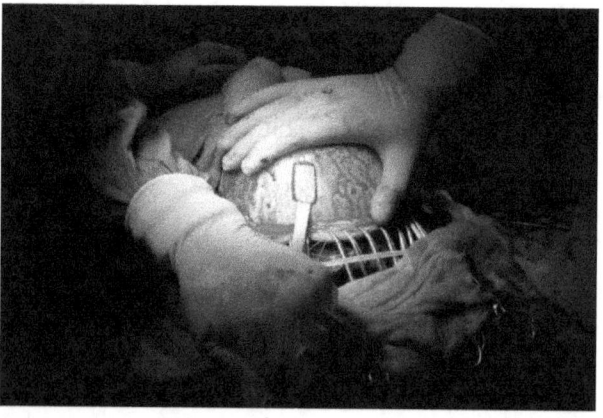

Figure 55 showing bicronal flap and bone graft for child to harvest in orbital floor reconstruction.

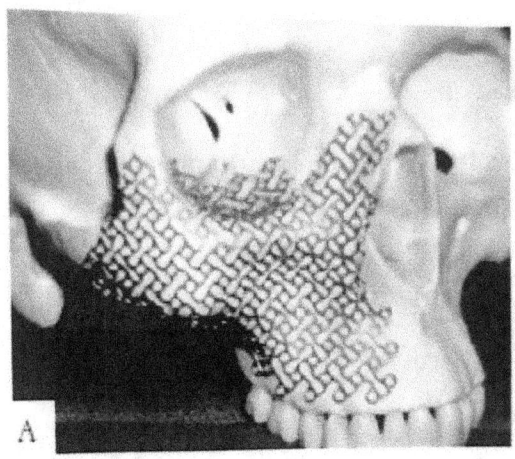

Figure 56 titanium mesh as reconstruction technique for zygomatic bone fracture and defect

Blow in fracture.

It is rare type of fracture result in inward buckling of the orbital floor.

It is orbital trauma and fracture of orbital floor and herniation of the maxillary sinus into the orbit through the thin bone of the antrum the (lamina paperchia) n the medial wall or herniation of the brain contents into the orbit we may be exophthalmos of the feature of blow in fracture and oedema, ecchymosis within and around the orbit.

Subconjunctival and circumorbital ecchymosis, diplopia, paraesthesia in infraorbital nerve, decrease in the volume of orbit and increase in orbital content (this is inverse to blow out fracture).

Chapter Six

The nasal bone fractures.

The nose is the most prominent subunit of the face.
The nose can divide into subunits, dorsum, side, tip, alae, soft triangles.

The clinical features of nasal bone fractures

Depression or angulations

Periorbital ecchymosis

Epistaxis

Tenderness

Crepitus

Septal deviation

Septal hematoma

The classification of the nasal bone fracture

1.   Front injury

A-   Plane1 (the lower end of nasal bone and anterior nasal spine).

B-   Plane 2 (external nose).

C-   Plane 3 nasoethmoidal fracture.

2.lateral nasal injury

A-without nasal septal injury.

b- with nasal septal injury.

Markowitz and Manson have classified NOE fractures into three patterns of fracture. They are:
• Type I: single-segment central fragment
• Type II: comminuted central fragment with fractures re-maining external to the medial canthal

tendon insertion
• Type III: comminuted central fragment with fractures extending into bone bearing the canthal
insertion. Injuries are further classified as unilateral and bilateral and by their extension into other.
  anatomic areas

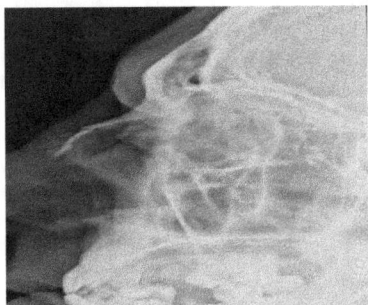

Figure 57 lateral skull view showing nasal bone fracture.

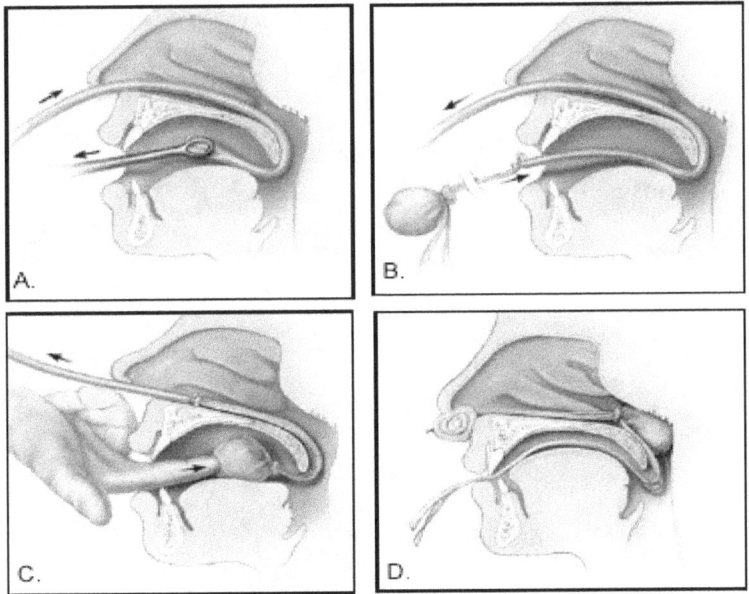

Figure 58 posterior nasal packing

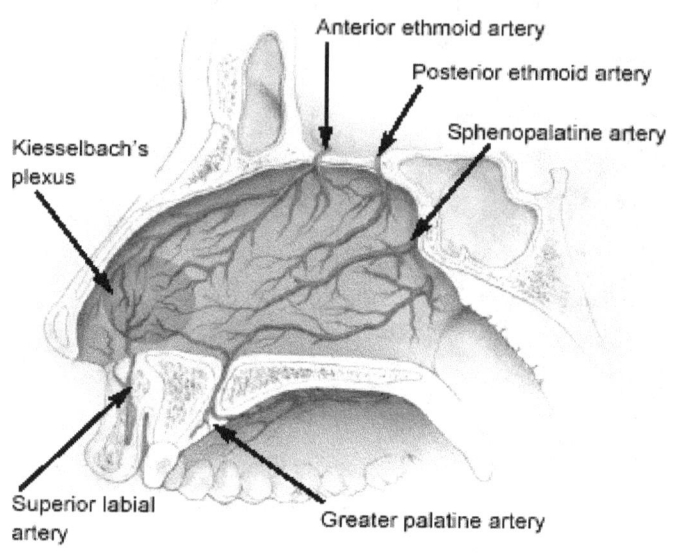

Figure 59 Kiesselbach's plexus form the blood supply of the nose.

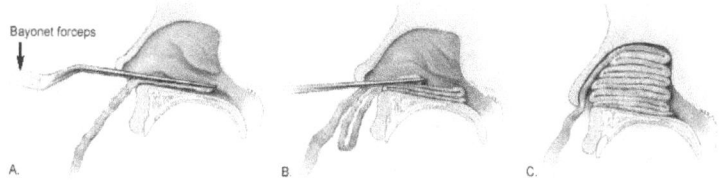

Figure 60 anterior nasal packing

The radiological examination

lateral skull view

CT Maxillary sinus.

CT facial bone

Treatment of nasal bone fracture

1. Reduction
A- Close reduction by manipulation by
   1. Walsham forceps for correction of the nasal septum.
   2. Asche septal forceps for correction of right and left nasal cartilages.

   Complication of nasal bone fracture

Saddle nose deformity is the concave appearance of the nasal dorsum that sometimes follows significant nasal trauma. It results from fracture and inferior displacement of the nasal bones, resulting in buckling of the cartilaginous septum and disruption of the upper lateral cartilage position. Late effects of the injury that amplify the deformity include septal collapse, which may result from septal hematoma formation, asymmetric septal growth, and scar contractures.

Anterior nasal epistaxis usually involves Kiesselbach's plexus, (Figure59) which is the confluence of the terminal ends of the superior labial, anterior ethmoid, and sphenopalatine arteries. Packing of this area with phenylephrine-soaked cotton pledges is frequently successful. Direct visualization with a nasal speculum may allow direct cauterization with either electrocautery or silver nitrate sticks to be performed. Excessive cauterization should be avoided, however, to prevent subsequent septal perforation. Most commonly, sterile petrolatum-impregnated gauze is carefully packed in a layered manner and left in place for 2 to 5 days. (Figure 60) Broad-spectrum antibiotic coverage should be initiated to prevent maxillary sinus infections caused by blockage of the middle meatus.

Posterior nosebleeds are more difficult to manage due to inability to provide adequate pressure with nasal packing. (Figure 58), this frequently is managed by placing a Foley urinary catheter into the affected nares, inflating the balloon with saline, and pulling the balloon back to seal the nasopharynx and to allow packing to be placed around the Foley. Tension is maintained on the catheter by placing an umbilical clip on it at the entrance of the nose. Commercially available posterior nasal balloons are also available.

Frontal bone fracture

The frontal sinus is absent at birth, but its growth is complete at about 15 years of age in most individuals. As a result, fractures of the frontal sinus are less common in children than in adults. The anterior table is thicker than the posterior one and more resistant to injury, and that is why it requires greater force to fracture than any other facial bone.

her frontal sinus is lined with pseudostratified columnar ciliated respiratory epithelium covered by a layer of mucin. Some authors theorize that the frontal sinus drainage is impaired after the nasofrontal duct becomes damaged or obstructed because of frontal sinus fracture.

These fractures are uncommon fractures (5% to 15% of all maxillofacial ones) with a preponderance of male patients aged 20 to 30.
the frontal sinus starts at birth and begins to appear as a pneumatic expansion at age seven from the nasal cavity, with complete development by ages 18 to 20.

classification of frontal sinus fracture

Type 1: Fractures of the anterior wall
1. Isolated to anterior table
2. Accompanied by supraorbital rim fractures
3. Accompanied by nasoethmoidal complex fractures

Type 2: Anterior and posterior table fractures 1. Linear fractures
• Transverse
• Vertical
2. Comminuted fractures
• Involving both tables
• Accompanied by nasoethmoidal complex fractures
Type 3: Posterior table fractures
Type 4: Very severe comminuted fractures of the whole frontal area, involving the orbit, the nasal base, and the ethmoid—Through-and-Through Frontal Sinus Fracture
The clinical feature of frontal sinus injury
lacerations, contusions, or hematoma welling, edema, or hematoma. Supraorbital numbness, subconjunctival hematoma, eyelid ecchymosis, and subcutaneous air crepitus and cerebrospinal rhinorrhoea.

Chapter Seven

Gun shot injury.

The classifications of gunshot injury
1.Pentrating injury it is a type of injury that the missile retaining in the wound, this is low velocity that missile embedded in the tissue.

2.Perforating injury the entrance of the bullet wound is small, and the exit of the bullet is large.

3. Avulsion wound it is the type of wound the soft and osseous tissues are destroyed with massive loss of tissue this occurs by bomb.

The causes of gunshot fracture
1.   High velocity missile, soft nose missile.
     Hardnosed copper jacket
2.   Low velocity missile shot gun is injury by airgun pellet.

The distance of shooting by gunshots are either: -

   1.Close range less than 10 feets.
   2.High range more than 10 feets.
   Dynamics of gunshot injury

   1.Military.
   2.Accedintal.
   3.Civil violence.
   4.Self-inflected.
The dynamic of the gunshot it depends on the velocity of bullet, the size and shape and extent of wound cavitation.
Soft tissues injuries
1.Contusion
2.Abrasion

3.Laceration

The site of wound
1.tangenital.
2.transeverse
Level of the wound could be: -
A. low, midlevel. high level of the neck.
The management of gunshot injury
A. Early management
B.
Advanced trauma life support
Primary survey
ABCD
(Airway, breathing, circulation, disability, and cervical injury)
Cervical spine stabilization
Neurological assessment
Secondary survey
Determine the extent of the wound.
Cleaning of the wound by betadine, normal saline
Removal of the foreign body
Wound debridement
Haemostasis
Closure of wound in layers by primary closure and gentil handling of wound and meticulous repair of the wound, not tied suture.
Pressure dressing 'prevention of infection by antibiotics and avoid sepsis.
Pain control by analgesics and pt follow up.
Late management of gunshot
Correction of the scar
Re establishment of bony framework including bone grafting
Reconstruction of damage nerve.

Soft tissue coverage (skin graft)
Special consideration of the face

1.. Lacrimal apparatus
2.. Facial nerve
3.Parotid duct
4.Commissure of the mouth
5.Eye canthi
Special problems in gun shot.

1.microsomia.
2.TMJ ankylosis.
3.Oroantral fistula.
4.prosthetic consideration.
Animal bite

Hemostasias
Debridement.
Approximate wound edges
Wound dressing.
Antibiotics and anti-tetanus vaccination.

Chapter Eight

Macq's

The answer in bold and black

Questions

1. Retrobulbar haemorrhage can lead to

A. **Blindness**

B. Diplopia

C. Proptosis

D. Blurring of vision

2. Miniplates used in fixation of middle third fracture based on

A. MacAfee system

B.**AO osteosynthesis**

C.champsy system

D. Fraulit system

3. Lowering the papillary of the eyeball occurs if

A. the orbital volume increase

B. **Detachment of suspensory ligament of Lock-wood occurs.**

C.   In case of blow out fracture

D.None of the above.

4. Maxillary artery most involved in fracture of

A. Mandible

B. Mastoid

C. Frontal bone

D. **Lefort fracture**

5. Which of the following is the characteristic of Lefort 1 fracture?

A.CSF rhinorrhoea

B. Bleeding from nose

C. Bleeding into antrum

D. Both and B.

6.Lefort 1 fracture is also called.

A. **Guerin fracture**

B. Subzyomatic fracture

C. pyramid fracture.

D. Green stick fracture

7.The battle sign in head injury indicated by

A. Orbital plate

B. **Base of skull**

C. Maxilla

D Mandible

8. In children below age 8 in Lefort 3

A. children in this age group get rarely affected by Traumatic accident.

B. Facial skeleton is covered with thick, soft tissue.

C. **There is lack of poorly developed ethmoidal and sphenoidal sinus**.

D. The of demarcation between medullary and corti-cal bone is less evident.

9.The tram line is seen in.

A. CSF otorrhea

B. **CSF rhinorrhoea**

C. The condyle mandibular fracture

D. in infraorbital rim fracture.

9.The pyramidal fracture has another name.

A. Lefort 1

B. **Lefort 2**
C. Lefort 3
D. None of the above

10. Blow out fracture of orbit involves fracture of which wall
A. Roof
B. **Floor**
C. Medial wall
D. Lateral wall

11.The most common cause of CSF leakage in middle third fracture

A. Frontal sinus

B. Tegmen tympani

C. Sphenoid sinus

D. **Cribriform plate**

12.CSF rhinorrhoea can be differentiated by all except
A. **High CSF protein.**
B. High glucose.
C. Tram line pattern.
D. beta-2 transferrin.

13.Gilles temporal approach for reduction of zygomatic arch fracture,
Rowe elevator is placed between: -
A. Superficial fascia and temporal fascia.
B. Temporal bone and temporal muscle.
C. **Temporal fascia and temporalis muscle**.
D. Skin and superficial fascia.

14.Hanging drop appearance on radiograph

A. **Blow out fracture.**

B. Blow in fracture

C. Nasal polyp

D. Nasal bone fracture

15.The nasal intubation is avoided in patient with

A. Maxillary fracture

B. Mandible fracture

C. Frontal fracture

D. **ethmoidal fracture**

16. which is not included in GCS

A. Eye opening

B. Motor response

C. Verbal response 1

D. Pupil size

17.the most common complication of rhinorrhea

A. Brain herniation

B. Blindness

C. Ascending meningitis

d. Cavernous sinus thrombosis

18. Which is not a feature of Lefort 2

A.   Enophthalmos

B.   Malocclusion.

C.   Paraesthesia.

D.   Rhinorrhoea.

19. Walsham forceps are used to
A. Remove tooth.
B. Remove root.
C. Clamp blood vessel
D. reduce nasal bone fracture.

20.parassthesia is common seen in which type of fracture

A. Sub condyle
B. Zygomatico maxillary
C. coronoid
D. Symphyseal

21. moon face appearance is seen in
A. Isolated Lefort 1 fracture
B. Lefort 2 and Lefort 3 fractures
C. Mandibular fracture
D. Isolated zygomatic complex fracture.

22. an average patient with maxillofacial trauma requires how much of daily sodium

A.100 mmol
B.50-60 mmol
C.10 mmol
D.1000 mmol

Further references

maxillofacial surgery Nilima anil malik

3. Textbook of maxillofacial surgery Kapoor

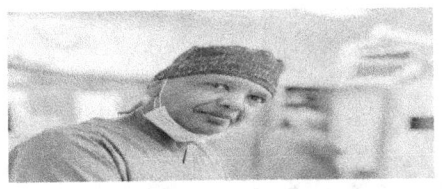

ABOUT THE AUTHOR
Dr. Adel Suleiman

Consultant oral maxillofacial surgery
Khartoum teaching dental hospital.
oral maxillofacial surgeon in
king Abdul-Aziz hospital Saudi Arabia
king Faisal hospital Saudi Arabia

BDS faculty of dentistry university of Khartoum
fellowship of oral maxillofacial surgery SMSB
fellowship degree Arab Board (Syria).

Another book for author

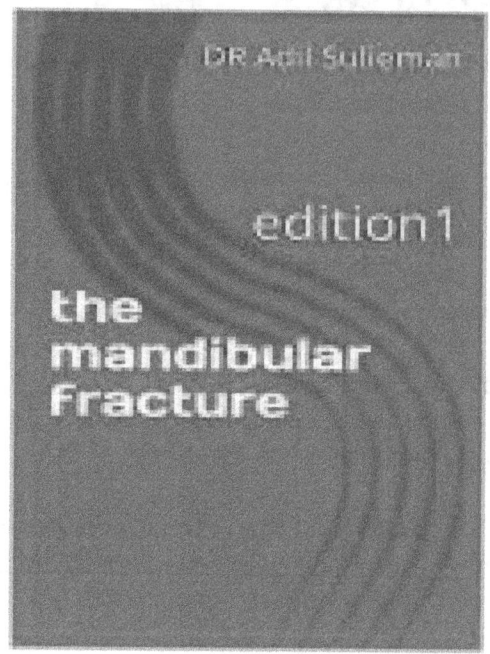

Network Site www.amozon.com

.

I